A Method
in the
Madness

Breandán Ó Seighin

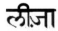

I would like to dedicate this book to all the dreamers, travellers and free thinkers out there. Never listen to those who say it can't be done, impossible is nothing.

CONTENTS

ACKNOWLEDGMENTS

I'm forever grateful to my parents for their constant love and support. Thank you to Liza Grantham for her patience, generosity and diligence in making the publishing of this account possible. To my teachers, doctors, nurses and carers for keeping me alive. To the people and culture of India: Sadhus, Shaivite, Tibetan and Ladhaki Buddhists, chaiwallahs and friends, you are always in my heart. To everybody I've ever met, fool or genius, you have contributed to this rich tapestry called life. The mountains and the oceans, planet Earth, bacteria and fauna, crows and monkeys, buzzards and vultures, the forests and the desert, as we are all one.

FOREWORD

Whatever your experience of mental health issues and drug use – be it personal, someone you know, or you work in this field – this account seeks to inform the reader of one specific case: the author's. It gives the background history, subsequent behaviours and survival strategies undertaken by the author who experiences an acute breakdown of mental health as a result of drug taking, and his bid to survive, prosper and function in an increasingly complex and everchanging world.

At times entertaining, yet sometimes surprising and shocking, the irregularities of mental health – however defined – and illicit drug taking are examined and explained in this book. Names have sometimes been changed to protect the guilty.

I do not condone or promote the actions in this book; it only serves as an observational account of one man's reality and journey through the last three decades and his struggle with sanity and life itself. The reader will hopefully find the given information useful to help people who deal with mental health problems or addiction on a daily basis, or to help with diagnosis, prescribing medication and tolerating certain illicit narcotics whilst avoiding others.

Let each reader take what they will from this account, some using it as a warning, others purely as a form of entertainment, amusement or a yardstick that could determine future behaviour patterns of people who suffer from health issues, addiction, or both.

Every case of mental instability or addiction is different, and therefore the use of the methods described in this book may prove helpful to some people but adversely affect others.

Providing such information will hopefully go some way to lifting the secrecy and ignorance regarding consumption of narcotics and their effects, leading potential or actual users to become more informed and in turn make better decisions regarding the choice of recreational drugs in the future. It may also serve useful to health practitioners or anyone working in the field of mental health when dealing with diagnosis and long-term care of patients.

1

EARLY YEARS

Nearing the end of a successful education, I was unwittingly introduced to cannabis resin at the age of seventeen. A joint passed round behind the garages opposite school between friends started an affair with mind altering substances which were going to change my life forever, with sometimes devastating consequences and at other times a source of inspiration – a beacon to follow, leading to many diverse adventures.

A happy innocent schoolboy, I passed all my exams with flourish, enjoyed sport, played music and was a popular, friendly, outgoing yet sensitive character.
I'd inherited a love of the outdoors from my father and was never happier than when in the Lake District, walking the hills, through forests and farmland, alongside crystal rivers and lakes, taking

photos with my Ricoh FF9 automatic camera of the beauty of this rural corner of England.

Having an Irish father and English mother, I experienced a conflict of interests during the Troubles years with very evident anti-Irish sentiment in England set against my love of Irish culture, especially the music, humour and the inherent beauty of the Emerald Isle, having memories of many happy holidays in rural Kerry during my childhood.

I'd grown up through the 70s and 80s bubble-gum years and enjoyed skateboarding and cycling in the street, climbing trees and playing in the fields and at the local park and tennis club. Idyllic innocence of youth yet meanwhile set alongside the turbulence and teething problems of immigration and racism, where cultures coexist and, inevitably, clash. Such historical events of this period included the Falklands conflict, football hooliganism, the rise of racist Skinheads, inner city riots, the miner's strike, the Birmingham Six, and the shoot to kill policy on the Rock of Gibraltar.

'There ain't no black in the Union Jack', 'No blacks, dogs or Irish' and the National Front were themes to be seen growing up in the North of England where people bought their vegetables on a Saturday from the town market, trailing round bored kids who would buy sweets by the quarter of an ounce with pocket money, all sold in paper bags. From the paper shop you could buy caps for guns, peashooters, Panini stickers and penny bubblies and get a job delivering newspapers if you had a bike.

I remember seeing punks adorned with pink Mohicans, rings and safety pins in their ears and noses, with a cigarette hanging from the jaw and nursing a two-litre bottle of cider. Only the watchful eye of a burly, handlebar-moustached police officer kept them in check.

My first experience of Asian cultures came when I visited the Tower of London as a young boy and saw a group of Indians, probably from Rajasthan, complete with white pyjamas and slip on colourful slippers that curled up at the toe. I found them fascinating, being so different to the bowler hat and brolly wielding Brit, reminding me of pantomimes and films such as Aladdin.

Visiting my Granddad, it was my job to go to the chippy for pie and chips while my mother cleaned the terraced house with an outside toilet. Later on, I'd be sent to buy Granddad's Benson and Hedges at a local corner shop run by Indians. Such corner shops were an overwhelming shock to the senses, with sights, sounds and smells never seen in a white middle class neighbourhood. Dark men speaking in different languages, dressed exotically, women in colourful saris, mystical music blaring out from a cassette player, fruits and vegetables of which I'd never seen the like, pungent and spicy smells that lingered on my clothes and me, about 12, buying two packets of fags for my Granddad. which I too was about to passively inhale.

Back to school on Monday brought more passive smoking as blue smoke billowed out of the staffroom and our wild ginger-haired teacher lit a pipe with matches as we copied our exercises from the blackboard and plumes of sweet tobacco smoke drifted around and encircled the classroom. It wasn't going to be the only time in my life I was mesmerised by matches lighting a pipe with the flickering flame dancing on the pipe bowl.

I was a cub scout which drew on much colonial heritage using the names of Rudyard Kipling's *The Jungle Book*, another introduction to native Hindu words such as Shere Khan, Baloo, Mowgli, Bandar Log, Bagheera and the like.

You have to recall that in these decades, there were three TV stations, now in colour! Everyone watched the same programmes, so you had common ground with playground chatter and games regarding Popeye, Donny the Bull, Stig of the Dump, Top Cat, The Wacky Races, Blue Peter, Jackanory, Morph in Take Hart, Harold Lloyd, Laurel and Hardy, Charlie Chaplin and later on our introduction to the USA through Sesame Street, CHiPs, the Six Million Dollar Man, the A Team, Nightrider, The Lone Ranger and Tonto and of course cowboy films.

There was no internet, no social media, no mobile phones and you dialled from a red public telephone box struggling to open the heavy iron phone box door and then tried to insert two pence coins as the pips went, or rang the operator to reverse the charges.

The rag and bone man came round on a horse and cart, the milkman came round for his money Friday nights who was also the tennis coach and the pop man brought Irn Bru and Raspberryade and you got money back on the bottles to buy more delightful carbonated fizzy sugar rush.

Such simple pleasures, but with teenage years came interest in the opposite sex, alcohol and music.

Along with friends I studied during the day, completed homework, walked the family dog, passed my driving test and worked on Saturdays in a supermarket, sometimes stacking shelves but usually larking about playing football in the basement.

Yet alongside this, I developed a habit for smoking joints every evening with friends or while taking the dog for a walk or a drag in the park. The hashish was often black Afghani, red or gold seal stamped with an Afghani seal, also known as Paki black, and Moroccan slate was also available. You'd be baked, euphoric, fucked, stoned, high, sometimes paranoid, happy, tripping, buzzing, excited... but if you tamed it, you could somehow function in this altered state. I developed a tolerance, so I had no problem driving or pretending to be normal to non-imbibers.

It was cheaper than drinking and didn't give you a hangover and meant you could drive your drunk friends around the pubs, skinning up in the car or the pub toilets and blazing one when you got the chance, in between pubs. It heightened your senses and you'd become more aware of music, vibrations and mood and at the same time forgetting the mundane as everything seemed more vivid: nature, clothes, lights and décor.

Add on top of this, when I wasn't driving, came countless pints of Guinness, Strongbow or Woodpecker cider, Malibu, Southern Comfort and combined with a live Ceilidh band or a Disco DJ in a nightclub and you knew you were in for a rocking night.

In the early years, you could overcook it and smoke too much or mix it with too much alcohol and have a 'whitey', which is defined here as nearly passing out and usually having to lie down, going pale, possibly vomiting but after a while you would come round and take it a bit easier next time on the substance.

Slowly other drugs began to appear on the scene and be experimented with. Speed (or amphetamine) parties during a six-week summer period left me wiped out in bed for a week and I never touched it again. (Also, it shrivelled my privates and I wasn't into that.)

Poppers was a craze that gave you a mad euphoric high for a few seconds and a pounding head – fun to use in the cinema, watching a cult classic like Easy Rider. It was sold in old seedy sex shops and was popular amongst the gay community. as it increased blood flow and relaxed the sphincter muscles.

The year I started smoking was 1989 and the vibrant music scene of Manchester was in full swing with acid parties, raves and the increasing emergence of electronic dance music. Coined 'the second Summer of Love', hedonism was all the rage, with bellbottom trousers, floral shirts, and a plethora of Indie music bands on the scene: The Happy Mondays, The Inspiral Carpets, The Charlatans, The Smiths and the Stone Roses. There was a revival of 60s music the Beatles, Jimi Hendrix and the Doors – the more psychedelic the better. Reggae music and of course Bob Marley, were also popular, as was Robert Nesta Marley's ethos of living,

My lifestyle started to drift from the mainstream, becoming more alternative, growing my hair long and wearing hippy clothes sourced from charity shops or the Affleck's Palace boutique. I had a girlfriend with similar tastes and I was accepted into a University in Birmingham.

The real meat of this account comes later, but in this first chapter I have to lay down the historical sequence and background giving the story some kind of perspective and at the same time a cathartic process for myself to put order where there has been chaos.

I completed my studies with a 2:1 degree in Business Management and the majority of my colleagues went into typically successful business careers. I enjoyed the course, mixing it up with playing football, pool and arcade machines, boozing every night and dancing, having the occasional romantic endeavour and, of course, smoking reefers.

Birmingham was, and still is, a cultural melting pot of friendly people having English, Irish, Indian, Pakistani and West Indian communities who, for the main part, live alongside each other peacefully for most of the time.

It was here I encountered Rastafarians, possibly second or third generation immigrants from Jamaica who sold sinsemilla (without seed) otherwise known as sensi, and sometimes harder stuff. Reggae music was big and the culture fascinating with its own language and street jargon, lifestyle, Rastafarian dreadlocks and apparent disregard for the law concerning illicit drugs. They represented an on-going struggle with poverty, discrimination and ill treatment by authorities dating back 400 years to slavery. This rang true to similar atrocities by the British when compared to their Irish neighbours and the 400 years of occupation.

It was in Birmingham that I was introduced to LSD and it blew my mind, having hallucinations and being transported to another dimension.

My first LSD trip with an Eton Old Boy, Sean, was a powerful magical experience. It was night-time and I was soon hallucinating on this acid and if you waved your hands in the air, trails would follow in the air better than any special effects in a film. Colours oozed and pulsated and we headed into a forest to ride the trip. The forest floor was a psychedelic carpet of intricate patterns, not unlike a snowflake under the lens, but in warm vivid colours and the whole forest seemed to vibrate and pulse as did my own body and mind. Tactile sensations were reduced so one felt no cold and impervious to physical pain, the drug releasing its power so a knock or a scratch would go unnoticed. I smoked a cigarette, which felt spongy and warm in my hand and could hardly feel the smoke going into my lungs, just a sweet warming sensation. Everything felt wonderful, alive and magical and I was completely in the moment, my mind being washed by the acid and leaving my thoughts and sensations new, fresh and childlike. As if in slow motion and at one with the nature, we wandered through the forest and came eventually to a children's playground and nearby bandstand in one of Birmingham's many parks. We were somehow communicating, Sean and me, when his face began to melt, the skin on his face just dripping off his skull so I looked away until this bad hallucination had passed. We kicked through piles of autumn leaves which glittered and shone and lit up, leaving hallucinogenic trails in the sky. The hallucinations lasted six or eight hours, losing total track of time and in a completely transformed state of reality. We finally reached the house and chilled on the sofa, coming slowly down off the trip with hashish. It was a good trip and, being the first, was a powerful mindblowing experience which would lead me to investigate psychedelics further.

Then came hallucinogenic mushroom picking and the powerful trips pushing my mind to the edge. We went to the countryside outside Birmingham and collected so many that when we pulled out of the car park, we hadn't closed the back doors of the van properly and they swung open and piles of mushrooms were literally falling out of the back onto the road.

Every weekend I would party it up, sometimes taking the train to Wales or Manchester, tripping in a forest, night walking and leaving the nightclub when things got too heavy. It was totally out of control and the odd bad trip would leave me fragile to say the least.

One trip, I had a fear and paranoia of being caught by the police: me and an old friend Tommy left the nightclub as the LSD trip was kicking in and wandered out of town to a local wood. I hid behind parked cars when traffic whizzed past, afraid of the police, but soon relaxed in the wood where we climbed trees and bowled through the forest, stopping to chat, smoke fags and skin up. Dawn began to break, and as we scaled a narrow ravine, a fox on the other side of the ravine, 20 metres away, stopped and fixed us in his view. It was a magical moment, totally in harmony with the environment and the fox stared at us without fear for which seemed an eternity, before it turned tail into the brush.

Later that year, I took a trip to visit Tommy who was allegedly studying the bottom of a glass in Newport. We had a wild weekend frequenting a venue called TJ's, where Courtney Love had played with her group Hole and Curt Cobain had supposedly proposed to her there. We spent the weekend getting wrecked and his young landlady (who was also his part-time lover) had some dubious contacts and I was sent into the chemist to get some dodgy prescription of uppers or downers for friends of hers who had a history of hard drug use.

I worked for a year as part of my degree for an International motor company but after such wild, colourful weekends, I obviously found the grey, no smoking office environment mundane, boring and irrelevant. But it paid well and I completed it.

After graduation, while most of my University colleagues were looking for work with reputable companies, I tuned in and dropped out. I signed on the dole and lived in between Moseley and Spark Hill on a street mainly inhabited by Asians, cycling round to friends in the alternative hippy scene there, going to reggae clubs and playing endless football games with Indians in the park in the summer. Balti curry houses were plentiful, good and cheap and I got a job delivering hire cars one day a week.

By this stage I was ingesting dangerous amounts of magic mushrooms and smoking hashish or marijuana daily. Living the dream, free as a bird or a tightrope to disaster?

Even now, I can't change who I am, nor do I want to, but I'm convinced life may have been somewhat easier and simpler if I'd never touched psychedelics and my mind might be stronger, although different, as a result. The same can be said for my addiction to joints and tobacco and alcohol, but in a way I've accepted those as my destiny: they make up a part of who I am today. I'm not here to judge, or be judged, for that matter.

All I know is that the capitalist corporate world reeked of wrongdoing to me, even before I took mind altering substances, being a lover of nature and the animal kingdom since I was a small child. And that will never change. I could never be the cut-and-thrust businessman after seeing the environmental damage and war mongering that multinational corporations and governments have done and continue to do. Reading the Guardian and giving £5 to Greenpeace was never going to be enough for me to quell my anger at how the planet has been polluted by commercial greed and toxic wars.

Once you choose a corporate lifestyle, you are part of the system and are trapped; unable to make decisions for yourself, as these company and government mechanised giants are on a highway to hell and seemingly impossible to stop. But that's not going to make me follow the crowd like a sheep, I may be crazy, I may be financially poor, but I've taken a stand and paid the price, and my conscience is clear.

If I want to plant a tree today, I just put my boots on and do it - simple as. I will not be told what to do by anybody, only guided by friends, love, spirituality and religious wisdom. That is why I refuse to have a boss, be it in the office or the home. I have to feel free to be influenced by nature, to be blown by the wind and sheltered by the trees so that I can aspire to live as far as practicably possible in harmony with nature.

Psychedelics push boundaries to what others may see as ideas set in stone, changing concepts of perceived realities, warping the concept of seen or unseen, allowing the user to see, feel and experience the sixth dimension and visions of the future. Of course, not forgetting they can also open a path to an intrinsic harmony with nature, providing a much bigger picture and overstanding of the cosmic oneness of everything.

In the 90s, I came up with an idea called the DVDream which would be a technology that would allow one to record dreams. Advancements over the subsequent 25 years means this concept may one day become reality.

Many people, through psychedelic drug experimentation or traumatic events such as military combat, are beset in later life by what are known as 'flashbacks''. Inadvertently, I created a method of dealing with such occurrences with a simple system I concocted to diffuse the negative and damaging effects such flashbacks could cause. I adapted the phrase "Random Play", changing its meaning from its CD music file origins and giving it a new, polysemic meaning, whereby random play referred to the mind freely presenting lived experiences or dreams from any given time, in no apparent order and without negative attachment. Accepting these thoughts as a perfectly natural condition, thus diminishing their impact on the mind, serves to relieve the recipient of the potential stress that they might otherwise cause. The same mind-control techniques, or tricks, are equally useful for combatting 'hearing voices'.

Some people's thought processes are different from others, some experiencing déjà vu, others dreaming, some having photographic memory. One of the earliest sensory memories I have is not an image, but an odour of a particular type of bleach or cleaning fluid that was used to clean a nursery I attended when I was two years old. Occasionally, often in public buildings, I get a match of the exact same odour and my mind travels back to my infancy where it recognises this smell from the recesses somewhere in my memory banks and reminds me that this smell is familiar and has been experienced before.

Humour is a great way of dealing with any given situation or experience. I find it hard to think of a situation where humour will not help one to accept any aspect of life, be it perceived as positive or negative. When one is confronted by a difficult challenge or threat, or has experienced a trauma or tragedy, with time, humour can help to digest and dissolve the negative impact of such an occurrence. Seeing the lighter side of a situation can reduce stress. If the situation at the time was positive or funny, then the humour surrounding it can be a constant source of positivity, giving one many a reason to smile, boosting happiness within and improving overall wellbeing.

Luckily, I'd travelled around Europe in my youth, having seen Mallorca, Amsterdam, skied in Italy and Bulgaria, Scotland, Ireland and Wales, but I fancied the exotic.

I'd thought about travelling outside Europe, possibly Chile, but changed my mind when some couple who had recently come back from India, convinced me it was the place for me. They were also selling good hash. Their tales of monkeys, adventures in the Himalayas, temples in jungles and special, cheap hashish sounded mystical so my mind was set on my next adventure.

2

CRACKS IN THE PLAN

Unfortunately, the wheels on my hedonistic lifestyle were about to buckle, unsurprising really looking back, but at the time I thought I was invincible, having all the vitality of a 22-year-old youth.

It had taken its toll. Drinking non-stop every night from my mid-teens and smoking weed since 17 and experimenting with harder drugs had inadvertently damaged my brain, not to mention my body. Wild nights of ten pints of stout, hell raising on drugs, dancing into the night and chasing women and music has a price to pay.

To this day, I believe all the factors played their part but I'd say the psychedelics of LSD and magic mushrooms were the key factor in my self-induced damage. Saying that, being short of stature at five foot six weighing in at 55 kilos didn't help as my drinking buddies were, in the majority, six footers and twice my weight, and we drank round for round.

In the January of 1995, I began to lose the plot, experiencing strange thoughts, paranoias and a confused perspective of reality.

I was convinced I was on some kind of mission, divine or whatever, and that it was my task to recruit a band of followers to change the status quo. I read signs from nature as a divine guide and was absolutely wild, sleeping rough, drinking anything and not taking any care of myself as I thought I was invincible. I thought I was some kind of Robin Hood figure. I repeat:

I believed I was a legend like Robin Hood.

Yes, I was convinced I was some kind of mystical legend with divine backing and unstoppable strength. Maybe that sounds amusing to the outsider.

God knows what my parents were going through, as this wild child roamed restlessly around, running through busy traffic, drinking in dodgy bars somehow avoiding confrontation, accidents or death. To this day, I don't know how, but what did I do next? I boarded a flight to India via Tashkent, Uzbekistan, on Uzbekistan airlines with a one-year travel visa.

3

HINDUSTAN 1995-96

This is the most unforgettable trip I ever took and it still holds a treasured part in my heart.

I arrived to hot and dusty New Delhi and was suddenly bombarded with a new world! The heat, the smell, the hot air in my lungs, Indians running around frantically here and there, shouting out in a foreign language and they were all the same size as me!

There was no dodgy vibe, no aggression, just a thirst for life and an overawing buzz of activity wherever I looked: technicolour chaos of movement and action, each with their own part to play.

I was soon whisked away out of hectic Delhi by a friend and took a train into the countryside. finally stopping at Orchha, Madhya Pradesh. A peaceful, lazy village lost in time, with simple farmers and traders eking out a living between temples and a palace fort with a beautiful river meandering by, surrounded by desert scrub with vultures circling overhead. If you've seen the Jungle scenes filmed in Cambodia for Apocalypse Now, with Dennis Hopper, then that's about how it was.

Here there was no alcohol or any need for it as the nature enthused every part of this village and me. The diet was yoghurt, small oranges and bananas for breakfast, peanuts, lentils, spicy vegetables, chapattis and rice for dinner. Small, bony sprat fish were sometimes available on the menu at the local fort, which doubled up as a hotel.

The locals went about their daily tasks, being merchants or of agriculture and running tea (chai) shops where the local young men gathered to smoke bidis, a leaf containing a very small amount of tobacco, played cards and drank chai. They spent the afternoon swimming in the river, hand washing their clothes with a bar of soap in the river, which they then dried on surrounding rocks while they soaked up the sun playing more cards and sharing cigarettes.

Days were spent swimming and chilling in the river, walking around the jungle and smoking *chillum*. A chillum is a clay pipe, which Indians use to smoke a mix of tobacco and charas, the name given to the special hand rolled hashish made in the Himalaya. It is a particularly strong resin with the hit made stronger as it is inhaled deep into the lungs through the chillum giving an explosive instantaneous euphoric effect.

With cries of 'Boom Shankar' by the locals and travellers alike, you are welcomed into a drug taking sect that has its roots in thousands of years of devotion to Hindu gods, particularly Shiva.

Yeah, man the Beatles were here! Tracing the steps of George Harrison never felt so good and I felt at home straight away in this Disneyland for hippies.

As for my delusional thoughts, amazingly, they just melted away in the apparent bliss of this dreamy landscape and stress-free lifestyle – uncanny, but true. The alcohol had been making me mad, triggered also by hallucinogens, yet the charas had a calming and uplifting effect on my sense of being.

The peaceful energy of this devoted Hindu society who were vegetarian or vegan and, in the majority, alcohol free, abiding by Hindu scripture and rituals, absorbed my apparent insanity, negativity and tortured soul.

4

VARANASI (BENARES)

We took a train to Varanasi (or Benares to give it its proper name), which lays claim to being the world's oldest city. Arriving just in time for the Holi festival of colour celebrating the birth of the universe, the place was electric with excitement, with people throwing paints over each other, throwing fireworks and partying to excess. The taxi driver had to make a few detours and U turns to avoid throngs of crazed men, wild on intoxicants, who menaced the streets in search of women and yes, it did feel quite unsafe. The atmosphere was at fever pitch and it looked and felt like a riot, as everyone was high on alcohol and *bhang* marauding the streets. Apparently it is the one day of the year that the city is lawless, which I couldn't quite fathom.

Many pilgrims visit this religious site, being on the

banks of the Ganges, and many come here to be cremated, believing it to be an auspicious place for determining their next incarnation. The city has a rich cultural and musical tradition with masters of sitar, bansuri and tabla based here. The ghats come alive with worshippers at dawn and dusk, as the funeral pyres burn constantly, with cows, water buffalo, crows, dogs and vultures adding to the jamboree. And through all this, the now placid Ganges flows eastwards carrying half burnt bodies and embers of the dead while freshwater Ganges river dolphins can be spotted occasionally in the murky waters. Having poor eyesight, they use echolocation for navigation and hunting, and somehow survive these polluted waters, often jumping out of the water displaying their prowess.

We sat with sadhus at night, perched on the Ghats, overlooking the river holding the moon's reflection and smoked chillums. One ascetic there did something which I still can't properly explain. I don't know what Jedi mind trick, hypnosis or magic he conjured up but it gave me an insight into the mysticism and power some sadhus are alleged to have after years of intense strict meditation, fasting, and devotion to yoga – breathing and training the mind to be at one with the soul and the heavens.

We were conversing in broken English with this wizened old man, when his glinting starry eyes locked on mine and I swear he read my mind and soul, looking into my eyes and entering into my body, deep down to my belly button I could feel his gaze penetrating my chakras and hidden soul and I was looking back at him, mesmerised and breathless, perusing his soul at will as if looking into space and back. To this day I can't fully comprehend what happened, but it was magical and only served to strengthen my belief in the mystic, miracles and faith in the unseen and the unexplainable.

The next day we tried balls of bhang, sold from the Government shops. Bhang is a crudely formed ball of cannabis which gives you a mellow trip, a dreamlike meditational state, often mixed in milkshakes to take away the harsh taste. It has been used in food and drink as early as 1000 BC in ancient India. Spaced out, you could observe dead bodies burn and smoulder while thousands of pilgrims on the ghats undertook ritual baths and ceremonies, drawn here by the Ganges and religious fervour, seeking temporary solace and release from hard lives, only to end in suffering and sorrow. The endeavouring spirit of fellow men, who continue on twisting paths of life despite encountering loss and heartbreak, never ceases to amaze me. Om Shanti.

So this is how I embarked on a wild journey around Hindustan, travelling by public transport, bus and rail, rickshaw and taxi, boat and coracle, and the odd hitchhiking with the lorry drivers, plus hiking and walking.

5

RAJASTHAN

The steam train puffed and wheezed sluggishly up over dusty dunes and undulating, unforgiving landscape as we ventured deeper into the Thar Desert, also known as the Great Indian Desert, the world's ninth largest subtropical desert covering an area of 200,000 square kilometres.

As a train lover, to ride a coal powered train of days gone by was a big treat, especially here, but the actual reality was a bit of a come down. It struggled to reach any kind of speed and dawdled along, and bits of ash and dust drifted into the compartment through the open barred windows which, combined with the heat, made me feel grimy.

The Nomadic Tribal people of Rajasthan contrast warmly to the harsh features of this barren desert landscape, wearing bright colours, playing wild music and travelling with camel caravans. There are the Kabeliya Gypsy people – the snake charmer caste – and Bopa Gypsy people who are musicians and singers depicting historical events and cultural facts that are passed down orally through the generations.

The older men wore traditional white pyjama suits called dhotis with red turbans and wizened brown faces, adorned with classic. curly moustaches, hands with geometric tattoos and whopping gold or silver earrings.

The women, not to be outdone, sported multi-coloured flowing robes with chunky metal ankle and wrist bracelets with bells, and intricately designed henna tattoos. This is an extremely hard existence, surviving and prospering in the harsh desert conditions and their resilience and strength is reflected in their colourful cultural activities of folklore, music and song.

I stopped a few days in Udaipur and saw the famous locations of James Bond's 1983 Octopussy with the Taj Lake Palace in the lake, Octopussy's home and the Shiv Nawas Hotel serving as 007's (Roger Moore's) hotel, but my main stopping point here was Pushkar.

A white city surrounding an artificial lake, Pushkar is strictly vegetarian and bringing eggs into the city is prohibited. Temples, ghats, boarding houses and rudimentary hotels dotted the edges of this murky water tank, which the Brahmins use to bless travelling pilgrims (and charge them in the process), who had come to pay their respects and take a break.

I got to know a group of travellers over the course of a few weeks there. They were quite unusual, being identical twins: two young French men who had hooked up with a pair of identical female twins, possibly from Canada, I can't remember now. But it was quite a spectacle to behold, being unsure if something I had ingested was making me see double. They and others in the group invited me to a party that night where there was music, dancing and smoking. Later on in the evening, someone offered me 'a line' to snort and, having only had experience of snorting amphetamine five years ago, didn't give it much importance or thought, and said "why not?"

Bholenath!! A casual slip of judgement and a case of mistaken identity was going to take its toll that night. What I actually sniffed, was brown sugar, a raw form of opiate, taken from the resin of the opium poppy plant, from which heroin is derived.

Unbeknown to me, the French male twins were young junkies and had come to India in an attempt to detox from the skag. but obviously weren't getting too far with that, not while I was there anyway.

Mashed, and with some other fools for company, we wandered the dark alleys of Pushkar coming to the Sun and Moon café where, in a semi-comatose state, lounged in hammocks, definitely on some other planet, puking now and then as is par for the course for initiates of such a drug.

I finally awoke in a white box room with colourful drapes, not remembering how I got there and, as the sun streamed through the window, everything felt pretty blissful. I sat on the doorstep, taking in the view as a cat woman from New Zealand did Yoga on the terrace of the room, which lead into an exotic paradisiacal garden of vibrant flowers, trees and bushes while peacocks strutted about, opening and closing their fans of feathers.

As if gazing on the supple, arching back and contorting positions of the young woman in front of me as she saluted the rising sun with her Yoga workout wasn't enough, the dazzling peacocks, not to be outdone, spread out there plumage to reveal a totally different but equally enchanting splendour. Boom Shankar.

The peacock's harsh and distinct call has comforted me ever since.

I was never to try brown sugar ever again (or heroin for that matter) and luckily never felt the urge or inclination.

I'd always had a fear of needles. At the age of six, I stopped growing for a year and was pricked and prodded by doctors taking blood samples and thus instilling in me a healthy phobia.

A softer option, drug wise, was to be had at the various bhang lassi stalls – some state-sponsored – where you could get a kind of ganja milkshake for a few rupees which kept you ticking over between chillums.

Finally. I moved on again, stopping at Agra to see the Taj Mahal, where the local Indians enthused over the rare sight of their city's freshly tarmacked road, only completed because of a recent visit by the current US

President Bill Clinton. The Taj was beautiful and impressive, as most monuments are, but lacked the pulsating energy I'd found in other, lesser known destinations in Hindustan.

My next port of call was to be Omkareshwar, in Madhya Pradesh, a prominent Hindu pilgrim sight at a confluence of rivers with an island in the middle in the shape of Om ॐ, hence its auspicious nature.

The pilgrims here were highly devoted, and a fervour of mystical energy surrounded the place, with temples blaring out cassette tapes of repetitive mantras (chants) of 'Om Nama Shivaya' from dusk till dawn.

With my old university friend, Charlie, we crossed onto the island to explore and camp there for the night. The flora was dry bush and the sun beat down relentlessly overhead.

We came to a clearing where at least sixty Langur monkeys were situated and it was just amazing. At almost three foot in size, the mainly white coats with a touch of coffee hue contrasted with black hands, feet and faces; they were truly wonderful.

They apparently posed no threat as we were carrying no food on display, yet some Indians had wisely brought various fruits and vegetables to offer them and some of the pilgrims carried staffs, probably just in case.

The next day, back on the mainland, we followed the river upstream where the rocks had been shaped and weathered by the riverbanks. One such feature were deep barrel size sink holes where pebbles, washed and spun by an eddying river current, had worn out these mini cavities when the river was at its height, probably at monsoon time.

Now with the river lower, these formations were interesting to see and in one we found a snake which had inadvertently ventured in, but now couldn't get out. By a placing a branch deftly inside, the creature could slither out and carry on its daily routine.

Further on up the river, we came to a small, but steep, sparse hill with a few trees and it was here I could see some kind of large animal in need of attention. On further inspection, it was a cow, which must have slipped and fallen down the steep embankment only to get itself wedged between two trees and couldn't free itself. What to do in Kathmandu? What to say in the USA? Que pasa en Mombasa?

We looked around for help but there was nobody else around.

Charlie was wearing a bed sheet (as he had a penchant to do in India) which he removed, and with it we created a type of harness and wrapped it under and around the unfortunate cow's belly. We then heave-hoed it, freeing it from its pincer-wedge trap, and lowered it down to the flat clearing at the bottom of the slope.

We got it to its feet, or should I say hooves, but I think the poor thing had at best strained or at worst broken one of its front legs and I think the latter was the case.

Not being able to help it any more we stood looking at the cow and its pathetic situation and eventually some local villagers came on the scene to whom we tried unsuccessfully to explain the situation to them as they responded by just nodding and shaking their heads.

Well, rescuing a cow, sacred in Hinduism, and freeing a snake, one of Shiva's adornments and symbols in this auspicious sight of Omkareshwar, you'd like to think brings some kind of blessing and karmic recompense. Ram Ram.

I frequented Gujarat and Rajasthan visiting popular tourist destinations, and finally made it up to the most majestic mountain range in the world, The Himalaya, the roof of the Gods.

6

ABODE OF THE GODS

This abode of the Gods was to be my home for a while and was a truly wonderful spectacle and environment.

Snow-capped mountains, oak, pine and eucalyptus; apple orchards, home to the amusing monkeys, bears, foxes, pine martens and suchlike, and the proud Himachali people.

I was based in Kullu valley in the state of Himachal Pradesh, home to sympathetic people who worked the land with sheep and goats, paddy fields and other agriculture, such as sweet corn and apples.

They span their own wool from the livestock to make lovely shawls and colourful clothes, giving the people there a distinctive, proud look and heritage.

The majority of homes didn't have running water, electricity or telephones, and there was no Internet or mobile phones at this time so it was a truly insular society cut off from the rest of the world.

A main cash crop here is the charas, with the best hash coming directly from this region.

Alexander the great had allegedly passed through here and legend has it that some of his soldiers stopped here to spend out their days. It's remarkable to see some people here that have blue and green eyes bearing testament to immigration of days gone by.

I stayed in the ancient town of Naggar at an altitude of 1800 metres and from here ventured to Manali at 2,050 metres and the hot springs of Vashist to where I another encounter with the ascetics of India known as sadhus.

Sadhus are wandering pilgrims who have renounced the material world and practice meditation, yoga and Ayurveda in order to rid themselves of the illusion of normal trials and tribulations of life and attempt to achieve Nirvana, an enlightened state. Doing so, they can determine their next incarnation.

Many smoke charas in devotion to Shiva observing rituals that have been formed over millennia.

I was to spend many a day with these sadhus who welcomed fellow pilgrims and travellers alike, sharing their time, knowledge, anecdotes, stories and humour (and sometimes bad temper) with whoever came along. In return, it's traditional to offer alms to pay for food or charas.

Their adherence to Gurus' demands can be extreme, having seen some who haven't sat down for 10 years, or who've performed other severe acts of penance such as forced solitude or going without food. Such actions train the mind to endure things we would normally regard as impossible.

It has to be noted that smoking charas in India can lead to unpleasant confrontations with the police, who use the law to extract money from would-be smokers, using the threat of jail as a bargaining tool. Baksheesh is the term used for this cat and mouse pay-out. It is advisable for tourists to always carry hard currency such as dollars on their person, to bribe such officials and avoid being thrown into a police station, and a possible jail sentence in some rat-infested hell hole.

I stayed in Vashist, renting a room in a simple, wooden guesthouse "upside", as the locals called it, perched precariously on the mountainside overlooking the village. I ventured into the village daily, enjoying hearty porridge and local honey to set me up for the day. I visited the hot springs and adjoining buildings which housed wandering ascetics who were sat cross-legged, round a fire – the sacred 'dhuni', which is a fire, smoking chillums and preparing food.

The hot springs were welcome and *very* hot, in contrast to the constant cold and rain as winter fast approached.

My appearance confused even the holy men who thought I was a female and shouted at me as I began to enter the male baths as there was a separate bathing area for women. I assured them I was in fact male, but it took some convincing, yet I was tempted and curious to follow their advice and bathe with the women! Bholenath!

The stonewalls around the baths were covered in moss and ferns and the baths themselves were open to the sky, where steam rose from these allegedly healing waters. Sat there in the hot sulphuric waters was bliss, soothing any aches or pains and I emerged renewed and cleansed.

The locals, in their white coarse woollen suits, had a custom of entering the hot pool fully clothed (which would cleanse them and wash their clothes at the same time) and then nonchalantly walked out into the freezing cold, absolutely dripping wet. I could only imagine that they would take days to fully dry off, unless they sat round a fire too.

Leaving the springs, the sadhus beckoned me over as, being obviously a tourist, I was easy prey for them to tax a few rupees off me. I was quite happy to spend time with them round the fire listening to their stories, songs, chants, advice and incantations to Shiva while we drank chai and smoked chillum after chillum. The art of smoking chillum has strict protocols in India when followed correctly. A thin piece of damp cotton is wrapped around the base serving as a cooling filter and the pipe is inhaled only once and then passed, to the right, round the circle of smokers until it is finished. Just before lighting, cries of 'Boom bholenath' and 'Shiva shambo' are enthusiastically intoned, paying respect and acknowledging one as a follower of Shiva, a Shaivite.

To the light the chillum, with matches, one has to puff on it a few times to get it properly lighted and only then inhale before passing it on, with the first and second hit being the strongest. The hit is instantaneous with a light headiness, kind of like an internal explosion in the head and a dizzy euphoria, and for several hours you can feel its effects in clear sharp vision and enhanced sensitivity to sounds. The body relaxes, the brain alert but in an altered state. You can converse coherently and it can bring a surge of energy so that you're able to undertake demanding physical exercise or endure harsh conditions such as extreme heat or cold.

A common stereotype in the UK of a weed smoker is of someone half asleep in front of the TV with munchies after smoking a joint, but here in India, the locals have always used it as a stimulant. Truck drivers who drive dangerously long 24-hour shifts on the hazardous roads here, often smoke or ingest charas or some form of ganja to keep awake. It can also open up the individual's creativity, becoming more open and perceptive to the otherwise unknown. One can focus more easily on the task in hand, particularly if it requires concentration, such as crafting gold jewellery or playing a musical instrument. Of course, like all intoxicants, different people are affected in very different ways. (A crude example of this is alcohol: some people will laugh and dance, whereas others will turn aggressive.) THC is not for everybody by any means and drugs don't suit everyone.

The chillum is meticulously cleaned after each use by threading a thin piece of cotton through the chamber of the pipe and rubbing it clean of tar and residues till it shines clean, as is the stone which fits inside the chillum chamber.

At Vashist, I was informed that some local ski slopes were open, North of Manali, not too far away, so I caught a bus as far as I could go before the road was impassable and walked the rest of the way through deep drifts of snow. Eventually I came to a very rudimentary ski resort. Solang Valley ski station, at 2,560 metres above sea level, was just a cluster of wooden huts, a couple of chai shop-cum-restaurants and one small ski lift. But in its simplicity lay its beauty and tranquillity. and I spent a few days trudging up the mountain and snowboarding down, in equipment which was broken and unsatisfactory (but I had a great time).

The sun was warming during the day and I would stop for a vegetarian hamburger and finger chips (French fries) and a bottle of Coca-Cola before returning to the slopes. Getting a chance to ski in the Himalaya was amazing, as I'd never had the chance to ski since my schooldays, when I went to Italy and Bulgaria. Here I was in my element. I met some other like-minded travellers and, after climbing the slopes, we would smoke chillum and then snowboard down the mountain. I must admit my snowboarding skills were limited and I regretted not hiring skis instead, to which as I was more accustomed and more in control on the slopes.

Night times were cold, and I'd sleep by a small, wood-burning stove in a sleeping bag, waiting for sunrise. Heavy falls of snow, sometimes up to two metres in one night, indicates the altitude and extreme climes of these mountains. One morning I opened my door to a wall of snow and had to climb out of the top of the door.

The few days spent here were very enjoyable and precious to me.

On returning to Naggar, I fell into a routine of smoking chillums every day, wondering and wandering the mountains of the Himalaya, playing chess with the locals and listening to Indian classical music on cassette. I rented a stone based, wooden, two-storey house with one room and a wooden veranda, set two kilometres from the village in lush vegetation and forest. I took many a walk, exploring the countryside and deep forests, never happier. The view from the balcony on the upper deck swept for miles down through paddy fields, orchards, forest and mainly wooden dwellings to the river Beas in the Kullu Valley, and then steeply climbed up the other side of the valley floor with similar landscape on the other side.

Above the orchards began the pine then oak forest line, followed by rough grassy pastures leading to sheer, rocky and finally snow-capped outcrops and massive mountain ridges. These peaks dominated everything around holding a powerful all-encompassing energy and aura that man could never come close to achieving. Truly majestic in their existence, no denying their prowess, invincibility and strength on a sheer scale and size that are difficult to comprehend; meekly viewed, yet somehow registered in the mind, and accepted as being all powerful, untouchable and existing. The mountain IS. The mountains ARE.

The views of the Himalaya and the surrounding valley were breath-taking, and to watch the sunset and the moon rise and fall over these white glistening peaks is difficult to describe, the awe they bring to the observer leaves one speechless.

The night skies were equally impressive with little light pollution: incredibly starry nights with shooting stars and satellites, and the moon, when full, lighting up the snowy ice caps and seemingly rolling along the mountain ridge.

During the peaceful days, I loved to watch the monkeys' antics; the locals weren't so fond, as they could destroy an orchard crop within a matter of minutes. I saw one such troupe and they scaled the apple trees in the orchard and instead of taking one apple and eating it whole, they would take an apple, take a bite out of it, throw it away and repeat the process, hence creating a destructive carnage for the farmer's crop!

Although my mind was calm, I had stomach problems, contracting giardia several times, a nasty parasite which induces stomach cramps, diarrhoea and feeling awful. I got it through contaminated water or food, and it's cured only by powerful antibiotics, a truly unpleasant experience from which my digestive system never truly recovered. It is commonly referred to as Beaver Fever in the USA.

I took two major trips from Naggar base camp, one to Parvatti valley, specifically Malana and the other, an unforgettable journey through Ladakh.

7

MALANA

To reach Malana, I had to trek straight up the mountain from Naggar at 1800 metres to Chanderkhani Pass, at an altitude of 3660 metres, where I camped for the night. It was tough going as I had the squits, still suffering from giardia. From there I descended down the other side of the mountain to reach Malana, situated at 2652 metres above sea level, isolated from the rest of the world with the peaks of Chanderkhani and Deo Tibba shadowing the village.

The economy of Malana was traditionally based on making baskets, ropes and slippers from hemp, and marijuana had been a legal cash crop for centuries. It is famed for the highest quality of hashish in the country and is known as Malana Crème and boy, sure is sweet. Bholenath!

The people of Malana have their own language and claim to be the oldest republic democracy in the world. They refuse to touch outsiders physically, and money has to be left on a counter before the merchant will then pick it up. Yes, we got very stoned here.

It makes me laugh sometimes when I see hill walkers with all the latest gear from Northface or Karrimoor going walking in the park. My mountain guide was something else. They are a true mountain goat breed. He had handmade stitched up shorts, an old pair of flip flops and some nondescript threadbare jumper and, on top of that, he was carrying a 40 litre plastic tank of illegal liquor, some kind of apricot moonshine, on his back with rough hemp rope for straps and he literally skipped up the mountain! Remember we are well over three times higher than Scaa Fell pike here, at 3,660 metres above sea level: this guy's in flip flops and I'm in some Nylon boots and kungfu trousers, smoking a pipe while "Commando" is getting shitfaced on hooch.

My Indian friend, Commando, got so drunk on top of Chanderkhani, the morning of the descent, he literally slipped, swayed, laughed, fell and staggered down to Malana, luckily with nothing broken!

Such style and snobbery in the Lake District makes me laugh, there wasn't a sniff of Gore-Tex in sight. For my 21st birthday, 1993. I took a group of students to Borrowdale near Keswick and planted a ganja flag on Hardcastle Crags while coming up on LSD, I think the acid was a penguin type. A passer-by, a nice man, obviously an intellectual, referred to the Cannabis Sativa flag and was at the same time curious and complimentary.

While in Malana there was a colourful village festival and they sacrificed a few goats and fed the people a kind of gristly broth or stew.

8

LADAKH

The second major trip was to the majestic Hidden Kingdom of Ladakh, formed when the Indian subcontinent tectonic plate crashed into the Eurasian plateau, forcing the original seabed up to 5000 metres, leaving a spectacular scenery second to none on the planet.

To reach the capital, Leh, I had to take the bus to Manali and then proceed by another bus on the arduous two-day ride over high mountain passes which are cut off from the outside world, the road only open for a few summer months, and the only other way in is by plane.

I nearly missed the bus in Manali and saw it heading out of the bus depot so I ran after it. Luckily, there was a ladder on the back of the bus which I jumped on, and climbed up onto the top of the bus with my backpack. I was greeted warmly by fellow travellers perched precariously on the roof. I do my own stunts.

Riding rooftop in India is enthralling, but you have to be constantly aware of low overhead electricity and communications cables. and be ready to duck unless you want garrotting.

There were some Austrians handing round the peach schnapps to warm the cockles as the bus was climbing to a very high mountain pass called Taglang La at an elevation of 5,328 metres, and the weather was coming in. I returned the offer of goodwill and passed round the fresh charas chillum peace pipe.

Ladakh is the highest plateau in India with much of it being over 3,000 metres (9,800 feet.). It extends from the Himalayan to the Kunlun Ranges and includes the upper Indus River valley.

The mountain ranges in this region were formed over 45 million years ago by the folding of the Indian Plate into the more stationary Eurasian Plate. The drift continues, causing frequent earthquakes in the Himalayan region. The peaks in the Ladakh Range are at a medium altitude, close to the Zoji-la (5,000–5,500 metres or 16,000–18,050 feet.) and increase toward the southeast, culminating in the twin summits of Nun-Kun (7000 metres or 23,000 feet.).

Ladakh's scenery is barren yet extremely beautiful and enchanting, with turquoise crystal lakes, large glaciers, colourful, rocky mountains in green, pink and orange hues, totally devoid of vegetation, and clear blue skies in the summertime. It is a desert, broken only by small green oases of villages with crops and trees. The residents are Tibetan, following the Mahayana tradition, and are a proud, hardy race surviving in extreme conditions. They speak Ladakhi, and Ladakh is dotted with Buddhist monasteries in spectacular locations. To break up the 48-hour rickety bus ride, I had my Sony Walkman and had happened on a series of albums called Soundscapes, with the Music of the Deserts by Zakir Hussain being my favourite.

With spectacular views from the bus, we meandered through beautiful high peaked valleys in surreal moonscape with the wonderful sounds of Indian exotic instruments, with their haunting song and beats. I found a comment on one of the tracks entitled Nomads a few years ago on YouTube that sums up the music of Zakir Hussain.

"This music takes me to another dimension, to my childhood, to a world beyond, to a sadness quite inexplicable. Phenomenal."

Siriam.

I stayed in Leh with a local family and spent the days discovering the bazaars and drinking a delicious local non-alcoholic beverage called tsetsa lulu juice, made from sea buckthorn berry, a bush grown in the area.

I hooked up with some Australian guy who was well over six-foot-tall, with a very pale complexion and long, flowing ginger hair. He chuckled as he told stories of entering remote Indian villages on foot and the villagers coming out, greeting him with awe, thinking he was Jesus. The Messiah has come!

The lady we stayed with cooked us lovely traditional food such as momos: home-made apricot marmalade and bread, and hot flasks of milky chai.

I hitchhiked deeper into Ladakh stopping at Lamayuru and finally reaching Rangdum Buddhist monastery, 4,031 metres, belonging to the Gelugpa sect on the edge of the Zanskar region. A remote valley, Suru valley is about 25 kilometres m from the Pensi La pass that leads into Zanskar.

I stayed there in the monastery a few days, again with giardia, and was delighted by their good nature and friendliness, their mystical chanting, rituals and music – the most impressive being the deep sounding call of the massive Tibetan horns. Tsultrim Allione described the sound:

"It is a long, deep, whirring, haunting wail that takes you out somewhere beyond the highest Himalayan peaks and at the same time back into your Mother's womb."

The snow was coming, so I had to leave before I was stranded there for the winter. I hitched out on a truck back to Leh and then headed on another long bus journey, not back to Manali but across to Srinagar, Kashmir.

We had to stop overnight in an army camp, as the road had washed away which was an experience in itself. The Top Dog (some Colonel or other) took a shine to me and let me sleep in his private quarters, unbeknown to me that his good nature wasn't all that it seemed.

I have to explain here that, throughout India, I had long flowing chestnut brown-blonde hair, and no stubble to mention. The Indians were constantly confusing my sex and mistaking me for a young woman, often with unfortunate, undesirable consequences.

So, imagine my delight on this makeshift army base near the line of control where India meets Pakistan and China, when I awoke to the Colonel's hand sliding up my leg in my sleeping bag! Luckily, the family jewels were untouched and I got him to behave. With so many men on that army base without a woman in sight, I don't think it mattered what sex I was!

Next stop was Kargil, which was a really edgy, vibey place on the Line of Control, very near to Pakistan. Basically, a transient army town connecting Srinagar with Leh, teashops had pictures of Ayatollah Khomeni on the walls and there was a despondency to the place. Four years later, there was the brief Kargil war and skirmishes between Indo Pak forces, with Pakistani forces eventually retiring.

I decided to visit a barber here and cut off my dreadlocks as they had become unwieldy, tangled and messy. The cut-throat razor was a bit of a shock and I think it was the most traumatising haircut I'd ever had, as people crowded round the shop to watch the spectacle. What a feckin' circus that was.

I eventually arrived in Kashmir which, although a popular holiday destination since the empire, was also tense due to conflict and sectarian disputes. I stayed on a wooden houseboat on Dal Lake with a Canadian girl I'd hooked up with. It truly was idyllic, but I was restless there, not helped by the fact that the Canadian girl had had a liaison with the Indian boy whose houseboat we were staying on months before.

It was pretty awkward, as he served up our meals, still holding a candle for her.

From there we headed on through the Punjab, stopping at the Golden Temple revered by Sikhs, and then back to Himachal Pradesh, this time staying at Dharamshala, home to His Holiness, The Dalai Lama.

A lovely wooden Tibetan refuge clinging to the mountainside, deep in India, it was given to the Tibetans by the Indian government. Unfortunately it is situated on a fault line and was the scene of a devastating major earthquake in the Kangra valley in 1905, measuring 7.8 on the Richter scale and killing 20,000 people. The most recent major disaster was in nearby Nepal in 2015, when an Earthquake struck with the same intensity, killing 9,000 people and injuring 22,000.

But here, life goes on, as the Tibetan community survives, apparently oblivious to this threat, or preferring it instead of Chinese persecution and extermination back in their homeland.

The wooden tea shacks dish up momos, noodles and boiled egg on toast with Bob Marley blaring out and the cool, beautiful young Tibetans enjoying their liberation.

It was a beautiful setting and there was a harmony about the place with the Free Tibet movement in full swing.

One afternoon, after imbibing, I took a stroll down to some palace and had the stupendous privilege to see His Holiness, the Dalai Lama himself, being entertained and performed to by some young monks in an open hall. There were pilgrims there who had trekked over the Himalaya from Tibet to offer devotion and seek solace, security, spiritual guidance and wellbeing in his presence.

He was smiling, and exuding a happiness, peace and calm throughout the hall, with little or no apparent security. I still treasure this fortunate moment of seeing Him there, happy with his people.

Saying goodbye to Dharamshala, I ventured, alone, back to Naggar to see in the autumn and the apple and charas crop. Multi-coloured birds visited the orchards, vivid red, green and orange, the size of sparrows, swooping around in flocks getting ready to migrate to other climes. From here I made my way west via Lucknow to Rishikesh.

9

RISHIKESH

Made famous to the West by the Beatles and their Guru, Rishikesh, in the state of Uttarakhand was my next adventure. Here I met Tim, another astronaut amigo from my University daze. I arrived during the night and, as the bus meandered down the winding road on the steep hillside, the scene was almost apocalyptic as brush fires were burning all over the surrounding hills, as if entering some kind of hell. The mountains glowed red and orange, sparking and smoking with intensity, and I was never to know the cause of such an occurrence, but at a guess, the fires may have been deliberately started to clear brush land by local farmers.

Staying at Lakshman Jhula, 5 kilometres upriver from Rishikesh, the pilgrimage boarding houses were simple and sparse, but cheap and full of other like-minded travellers with musical smoking sessions taking part throughout the day on verandas and balconies in sweltering temperatures overlooking the river Ganges (known as Ganga or Mother Ganga to Hindus). I managed a few tunes on a harmonica I'd picked up and other travellers had didgeridoos, guitars, tablas and the like but I smoked more on the peace pipe instead of playing any instrument seriously. I was too blissed out for that, just being, and soaking up the vibe, sounds, sights and smells, dreamily floating through this wonderful land of sensational surprises.

The ghats, or bathing areas were steps going down into the Ganges where people would come to wash, do laundry and ritually bathe in devotion. To bathe in the Ganges is deemed auspicious for a Hindu, remitting sins and can help a fortunate reincarnation or may help break the actual wheel of constant reincarnation, instead ascending to Nirvana.

The Ganges is a sacred river to Hindus along every fragment of its length. All along its course, Hindus bathe in its waters, paying homage to their ancestors and to their gods by cupping the water in their hands, lifting it and letting it fall back into the river; they offer flowers and rose petals and float shallow clay dishes filled with oil and lit with wicks (diwas). On the journey back home from the Ganges, they carry small quantities of river water with them for use in rituals.

The Ganges is a powerful river in a very physical sense also stretching 2,525km from the Western Himalaya to the Bay of Bengal.

At Rishikesh, the river surface appears flat

and smooth, hiding the depth, the sheer immensity of volume of water it is carrying and has dangerous rips and whirlpools. It is approximately 120 metres wide here and possibly 10 metres deep or more, depending on the season.

Unfortunately, swimming is not mastered by all Indians, and such a river presents a perilous challenge to even the strongest swimmers. Tim and I were drying off in the sun after a dip and were watching the river flow by. The following quote by India's first Prime Minister sums it up nicely:

> "Ever-changing, ever-flowing and yet ever the same Ganga."
>
> Jawaharlal Nehru.

The ghats were a hive of activity as day-trippers and seasoned pilgrims alike took to the waters and a large footbridge suspended half a mile down river was thronging with people coming and going across the river.

A young family about 40 metres away had been partaking in this ritual until catastrophe struck. Somehow, one of their young children either fell or got swept into the river, into the powerful currents of the Ganges and the mother started screaming and shouting which rippled down the bank as other people tried frantically and desperately to help. It happened very suddenly but I can, to this day, only assume that the people there were unable to swim or petrified of the water and so watched, as if frozen or helpless, as the child was carried away, soon to be pulled under, never to be seen again. Why no one had made a more concerted effort to save the child by jumping or diving in after her, I will never really know.

The whole bank of pilgrims were shouting and screaming and even people from the footbridge realised what was happening, joined in this desperate, oh so cruel, outage of grief and suffering. Tim ran down the ghats and dived in, to no avail, and returned despondent ten minutes later. I think everybody was in shock.

The ghats cleared of all people and suddenly became quiet, still and eerie as if the people were in fear, absolutely scared witless of this sacred river, its sheer overwhelming omnipotence. Indians are superstitious at the best of times.

As we sat there, trying to comprehend what had just occurred, the tragic, seemingly preventable loss of a sweet innocent life, there came a polemic mood shift from peace to despair, and the only noise to shatter the silence was a cry of a baby coming from across the river on the far bank.

What solace the parents could take from their religion regarding such a tragic incident, I couldn't begin to imagine. Death is when faith in one's beliefs are tested to the maximum, but Shiva is regarded as the Creator and Destroyer, one of the supreme beings who creates, protects and transforms the Universe.

The story behind the image of Shiva with the Ganges in his locks is that a sage told him that he could save his life by bringing the sacred river Ganga down from the heavens to purify the souls of him and his ancestors and help them to attain nirvana.

Shiva is All and in all, the creator, preserver, destroyer, the cosmic ecstatic dancer, Nataraja - Lord of the Dance.

From Rishikesh, Tim and I headed north in search of the source of the Ganges. We travelled North and set up at Gangotri, still in the state of Uttarakhand in the Uttarkhashi district, a rough town of wooden shacks and dwellings reminiscent of some gold rush wild west town. From there it's a day's trek to the actual source of the Ganga, which flows from a glacier at Gomukh.

We stayed a few days in Gangotri, allowing our bodies to adjust to the altitude, which is elevated at 3,100 metres above sea level, hanging out in chai shops and sleeping on rustic wooden beds with a blanket or two in rudimentary wooden abodes. The sun was welcome during the day as we investigated the town, its river, waterfalls and places of retreat, yoga and meditation. The river was especially powerful and turbulent here as it thunderously cascaded down the valley, pounding and cutting through the rock formations and the surrounding mountainous forest scenery was spectacular.

We made the uphill 19-kilometre trek to Gomukh at 4,023 metres close to the Tibetan border, entering into a rock-strewn, cold land with all the indications of a terrain formed by a glacier and glacial deposits. We were welcomed by the majestic Mount Shivling, its iced face and peak brilliant, shining and dazzling white under the sun's glare. There we met a sadhu by the source of the river who had a makeshift plastic tarp serving as a tent bolstered by dry stone walls. He welcomed us to stay with him and provided shelter, chai and rice and entertaining discourses.

Gomukh is the terminus or snout of the Gangotri glacier, one of the largest in the Himalaya with an estimated volume of 27 cubic kilometres from which flows one of the primary sources of the Ganges. It stretches 30 kilometres, the snout being at 4,200 metres and extending back up to 7,000 metres at the top where it begins.

To bathe here in the frigid waters spewing from the ice cave is considered auspicious and holy for Hindus, washing away sins. We bathed here in the icy waters, lucky not to catch hypothermia, and then joined the sadhu round a small fire in his temporary dwelling drinking chai, smoking chillum and conversing. He prepared us some simple fare of lentils and rice but having a sweet tooth, I pulled out a packet of sweet biscuits to crave my need for sugar but the Sadhu wasn't impressed and admonished me for my behaviour. I slept a broken night awaking several times uncomfortable due to the cold temperatures and rocky ground with only a cotton blanket to protect me against the perishing air.

The next day, we walked back down to Gangotri refreshed by chai and the warmth of the sun and after a night in Gangotri, we then headed to Ghuttu to start an eight-day trek to the Khatling glacier.

After staying the night in some lodgings at Ghuttu, we stocked up on food supplies in the village shop and began our ascent with only a rough map to guide us. The trek was mainly uphill as we ascended altitude through magnificent untouched mountain scenery and its valley, following the meandering river, indicating the way to the glacier, another tributary, which finally joined the Ganges.

We calculated that it was a five-day trek up to the glacier and a return journey of three days' walk as it was downhill all the way.

Forests were abundant on the slopes of the mountains giving way to sheer rock faces and huge, cascading, misty waterfalls. Clearings in the forests gave up lush green pastures for the nomadic herders to tend their flocks of sheep and goats who migrated downstream as winter approached, sleeping in rustic barns if available or beneath the stars, alert to any threat to the flock.

Predators here are several, including eagles, foxes, Himalayan black bears and snow leopards, as well as smaller vicious animals, such as pine martens and stoats. We crossed paths with some herders who were particularly interested in my Swiss army knife. Their clothes were made from the wool from spun from the flock; they would also kill an animal occasionally for sustenance, cooking it on wood sourced from the plentiful forest. They led a very simplistic existence, in harmony with their surroundings.

We slept under rock crevices at night and made a fire and cooked simple food, our rations running low not helped by some thieving crow that made off with our bag of sugar.

On the third day we came across a village totally cut off from the rest of the world, with crude wonky stone slate roofs hewn from the local rock faces and smoke drifting from the chimneys. The land here had been tilled to provide some crops and it really looked medieval. A couple of young boys meekly acknowledged us and one of them showed me some warts on his fingers and body, wondering if I had a cure. I happened to have some wart or verruca cream which I happily gave him, not really sure if it would do the job.

We stayed that night in a Government lodge there and enquired of the possibility of food but the man there refused. He actually thought I was Tim's girlfriend but a quick flash of my privates quelled his mistaken curiosity. In the end, he brought a basic camera he had somehow acquired. He didn't have batteries or film, or seem to know how it worked. I offered him both batteries and a 36-exposure film in exchange for nourishment so the deal was done. After what seemed an age he returned with a pot of spinach, some chapattis and goat's milk which had gone off and was fizzy and sour, but we wolfed it all down, nonetheless.

We finally came to the day we were going to reach the destination of the glacier, having traversed scree slopes and mountainous terrains, crossing rough, half rotten, wooden footbridges with the rushing waters close below and really feeling at one with nature. Tim was sick – I can't remember if it was the altitude or a stomach problem, but he couldn't go on, so I carried on alone so as to partake in seeing this untouched glacier in this oh-so-pristine valley.

Now on my own in this huge valley, I carried on walking for a few hours until I finally came across the view I sought of the Khatling glacier in all its majesty. It was uncanny that here, at 3,800 metres, in this vast valley, high as it was wide, I was the only human living soul within miles. I could feel the pulsating energy of such a place flowing through and all around me. As I sat there tired, yet in awe, I felt at one with the mountain, peeled off my boots and took it all in for an hour or so, ate a frugal meal, took a photo and then headed back down to my rendezvous with Tim in some abandoned stone shelters we had passed earlier that morning.

I came across animal prints and excrement, which looked like bear so I was constantly on the look -out and alert to any untoward encounter with a native of these parts. Happy to see Tim after my solitude, we made a fire and I smoked a chillum on my own (Tim had recently gone teetotal) as he read aloud from Jonathan Livingston Seagull by Richard Bach.

This had been a great experience and wonderful adventure not without its difficulties, but one I will always treasure wherever I am.

We headed back to Rishikesh and eventually bid each other fond farewells, wishing each other good luck for our coming separate journeys, and I headed down to Delhi from where I would venture south.

I was getting ready to escape the Himalayan winter and head down south to the other end of the Peninsula, via Delhi then first stop Kerala, only 3,435 kilometres away!

10

KURUKSHETRA

On my way down to Delhi, I visited Lucknow, the setting for Rudyard Kipling's book Kim. There wasn't much for me to see there, but whilst I was at the train station planning on taking a train to Delhi, I noticed a lot of pilgrims and sadhus on the platform and enquired where they were going. There was to be a solar eclipse and it coincided with a major festival at this deemed sacred place where the battles of the Mahabharata took place in the land of the Bhagavad Gita.

Every, year lakhs (hundreds of thousands) of people come to take a holy bath at Brahma Sarovar on the occasion of "Somavati Amavasya" (Sacred No-Moon Day that happens on a Monday) and on solar eclipses. They believe that a bath in the holy Sarovar frees all sins from the cycle of birth to death. The Sarovar is one of Asia's largest man-made ponds.

So, I decided I too would join the pilgrims and made my way by train to see this festival. I arrived at night and leaving the chaotic train station there, I donned my hood so that I could fit in with the pilgrims there and not attract unwanted attention. I boarded the back of a bullock cart full of travellers and having paid my fare, we trundled along the road and soon we were at the sacred festival site. People were everywhere bedding down for the night, sleeping below the stars around small fires. I bought some firewood and set up a little fire, smoked a few chillums and the stars were magical, and the hub bub of the pilgrims was with smoke drifting on the air made it a mystical medieval feeling.

While queuing to buy the firewood, some people greeted me and enquired where I was from and in broken Hindi, I replied I was from Nepal and they were calling me Nepali Baba.

It is interesting to note that I chose to go incognito at this religious festival. Later on in life I discovered that travellers in medieval times, who had visited Mecca and China, often travelled in disguise, otherwise their journeys would have been more perilous or, in fact, impossible. Spies on missions concerning the Great Game around India, Afghanistan and Russia would also travel in disguise to fit in with local communities and travel without restrictions, accessing locations that were strictly off limits to the foreigner.

The next day I awoke early and most of the people were up and about. I sourced some breakfast of chai and bread and wandered around this amazing site with people bathing in the vast tanks, sadhus grouped together round fires hailing Shiva as they smoked chillums. There were sadhus of all types and colours, some observing strict penance such as an arm raised for 12 years or not sitting down for an equal length of time and only sleeping stood up, leaning on what looked like a swing hanging from a banyan tree.

I got acquainted with one sadhu and we spent the time smoking and talking. He seemed ok at first, but when I expressed my preference to leave him the following day, he got a bit freaky and started following me, maybe as I had the best quality of charas to smoke and he saw me as an easy target to obtain money. In the end, I left but he started to follow me, and it was beginning to do my head in. I felt vulnerable and it was time to leave the festival anyway, and as I was crossing a bridge, the sadhu in pursuit hailed a policeman and informed him I was carrying charas. I told the policeman he was harassing me, and luckily he let me go and reprimanded the sadhu and I finally boarded a bus in the direction of Delhi.

The bus was hot and dusty, and I was physically and mentally drained, so I alighted the bus at Panipat, 90 kilometres north of Delhi and found a small park with shade in which to chill out. I didn't really know where I was at the time, but thought I'd let destiny lead my way and explore a place off the typical tourist map.

I wandered into the old part of the town and was walking down a small street where I attracted the attention of some kids who started to follow me and shout "Angrezi" which means English in Hindi. The group of kids began to grow, and I wasn't sure what to do, when an old man came out of his dwelling to see what all the commotion was about. He ordered the kids away and invited me into his abode.

It was quite a large building, very old, in a Mughal style with an interior square surrounded by grand ornate arches though in a poor state of repair. He lived alone and was happy to have company and somehow we conversed in my limited Hindi and he provided simple fare and chai to drink and offered me to stay the night in a charpoy bed, the classic bed found all over India. He showed me treasured photos of his family, now deceased, and was a very charming and humble gentleman who had obviously had a hard life.

Finally, he brought out a simple rudimentary clay pipe about four centimetres long, which cost a few rupees, and some very dry ganja leaves and offered me a smoke. I motioned for him to wait, as I rummaged in my bag and brought out a 15-centimetre polished fine chillum and India's finest charas, Milana crème. His eyes lit up and stated I'd been sent to him by the gods or something to that effect. He'd probably never in his lifetime smoked this best quality, sticky, dark brown charas and was truly delighted and over the moon, at the same time wondering how this strangest of strangers had arrived to bring him such a coveted smoke. He thanked and hailed Shiva as we shared a few chillums before thanking me profusely and then we retired to sleep. The Indian people readily believe in and accept the mystic, and he truly believed I'd been delivered to him by the gods. We parted a fond farewell the next morning, I left him some charas which he would treasure, and boarded the final stage of the bus to new Delhi.

Having arrived in Delhi a few times using it as a travel hub, I always stayed in the Pahar Ganj area with hotels and eateries set up to cater for tourists such as myself. It was there I met a colourful character that was a trained vet, maybe from Quebec or Germany, I don't recall. He had been unusually fortunate in that he had been given permission to live in the village of Malana and had been accepted by the locals there due to his veterinary knowledge. He solved livestock problems with otherwise unheard-of vaccines and medicines and I think he also acted as a quack doctor to treat the villagers. He was happy as he had a constant supply of the best charas in return but I don't know how long his position there lasted because the winters were harsh, the villagers very particular and he was probably a target for the local police as he easily stood out.

He'd been visiting Delhi and had captured a monkey that had been creating havoc in the restaurants in Pahar Ganj. It's teeth had been filed down so had obviously been used as a street performer in captivity and had escaped and lost its owner.

What the vet was going to do with this half wild animal, God only knows, but there it was in his hotel room eating cigarettes, of all things. It had been hooked on tobacco from its previous owner and then forced to perform in order to gain recompense of food and tobacco which seemed the only solution to stop it going wild and aggressive.

Such is India, one never knows what to expect next.

11

THE SOUTH

I've always loved travelling by train and in India it was no exception, in fact it was better than any other train ride I'd taken before in Europe.

The windows were wide open due to the heat as were the doors so you could sit on the footplate and observe rural India as the train meandered this way and that on this epic 54-hour locomotive journey from New Delhi to Kerala in the south.

After leaving the urban sprawl of Pahar Ganj, Connaught Circus and the capital New Delhi, the land became barren and arid and unforgiving. Villages were clusters of mud and cow manure cemented dwellings with straw roofs, with barefoot kids in colourful rags playing under the sun, skinny wild dogs roaming about while the people toiled the land and transported goods via cart and ox. Cows would wander around looking for anything vaguely edible be it pinched from a vegetable street vendor or a discarded cardboard box. The medieval conditions in which many people in rural India lived, never ceased to amaze me, an extremely hard life but handled with grace, composure and a certain dignity and more in harmony in the natural environment than any city dweller could pretend to achieve. The women dressed in saris or tribal dress and the men involved in farming also attired in traditional dress whereas the younger men were donned in trousers and shirt and the inevitable sandals or flip-flops.

Sitting on the footplate, smoking, watching a non-stop never-ending display of vibrant life in this huge country is second to none. The constant activity and display of peoples, livestock and wild animals is breath-taking as one attempts to take it all in.

A family washing under a hosepipe blissfully unaware of the lack of any privacy, people defecating in scrubland next to quagmires of polluted dark, toxic water. Egrets perched on the backs of cows and water buffalo or stalking insects in the fields. Squawking crows perched on a tangled spaghetti of telephone and electricity wires, monkeys de-licing each other atop apparently thrown up concrete dwellings or causing mischief, always on the look out to steal fruit and vegetables from street vendors who sell their wares from wooden carts pushed around on four bicycle wheels. Dreadlocked tribal urchins playing in the dirt, happily waving at the passing train. Kids knocking an old tyre or rusty bicycle wheel with a stick down a dusty track. Women selling their home-grown vegetables, sat down on the floor on a rug, haggling and bartering in a bustling market. Sadhus and locals seeking shade under a banyan tree, paying respects to one of the pantheon of Gods, smoking, offering alms, sharing tales or receiving advice or blessings. People taking solace and seeking shade from the sun in chai shops and restaurants dishing out spicy thalis with rice, daal, chutney and curried vegetables. Taxis, auto rickshaws, buses, Ambassador cars, mopeds and motorbikes and the garish brightly painted trucks all fighting for space on the highways and byways with little sense of order, only the sound of blaring horns giving precedence or right of way, black and blue fumes billowing out behind while cows sleeping in the roads seemingly nonchalant and unaware of the hustle and bustle yet perilously situated. Temples blaring out mantras through loudspeakers, and the competing mosques with their call to prayer. A criminal being frogmarched down the road by police with a rope around his neck, just to be sure he doesn't escape. People chewing betel nut, spitting long trails of red saliva on to the dusty earth with red eyes to match from the intoxicants in this popular fix. Hand painted billboards of Bollywood's latest offering, Pepsi, Coca-Cola or Thums Up, a fizzy drink, or the local STD clinic or advertising a miracle cure for lack of libido or premature ejaculation. Mechanics, black as oil, working on wrecks of chassis in the street and horse drawn cargos precariously balanced with seemingly unjustifiable loads of hay or sugar cane. Young men holding hands to show the strength of their friendship, sharing cigarettes, drinking chai, chatting and laughing and playing cards. During the light of day, this country never stops. People everywhere going about their daily tasks and duties making India a vibrant society and culture, which is a wonder to behold.

The next day, having left the arid capital and its surrounds, I awoke in the train's three-tiered sleeper compartment to a totally different scene of dense tropical lush vegetation, palm trees and lagoons and a humid sticky heat.

Having traversed the length of India, passing through different climate zones, you could mistake yourself for being in a totally different country.

Lagoons and backwaters with boats sleepily cruising along, towering coconut laden palm trees next to whitewashed temples and walls adorned with the hammer and sickle.

It was humid and the landscape was totally different. Even the people looked different, of darker complexion, and with the trademark *lunghi* (similar to a sarong) a folded brightly checked cotton material worn just above the knee.

The south has its own particular distinctive cuisine as well: idlis, masala dosas, and a rich variety of ingredients for the thaliplate or curries due to the tropical surroundings- coconut, jackfruit and other such exotic fruits and vegetables.

Known as the Malabar coast, this area has been trading in the exotic for thousands of years and been a trading hub from east to west, even predating Roman times. Throughout recorded history from about 3000 BC, the Malabar coast had been a major trading centre in commerce with Mesopotamia, Egypt, Greece, Rome, Jerusalem and the Arab world, this trading route known as the Spice Route, linking

India with the Old World.

Wonderful fresh fish from the Arabian Sea continues this trade and rich fishing heritage and industry along the coastline where villages sell kingfish and shark, lobsters and prawns and many other types of fish and seafood from the restaurants, tandoors or beach shacks. Coffee here is very popular, as is fenny, an alcoholic spirit made from cashew nuts, sold in cheap portions of small plastic sachets from dowdy government shops to tipplers, boozers and alcoholics alike.

It seems the Government's hand was forced into providing this service as locals were producing their own hooch, which at times was so strong, it was making the consumer blind!

The tropical blue skies only met there match as sunset approached with vivid orange, maroon, purple and red skies which seemed at time inflamed with such intensity, they could set alight the land in some kind of Biblical occurrence.

From Kerala, I meandered north, up the coast to the neighbouring state of Karnataka, specifically to the village of Gokarna, a Hindu pilgrimage destination with several idyllic unspoilt beaches with only beach shacks to compliment the view. The villagers were merchants and fisherman and Brahmins attending the Temples and religious festivals held here.

Om beach, given its name as it is in the shape of Om ॐ is hence auspicious and sacred. This was where I chose to stay for many months in the winter, baked on the beach by the sun and the chillum.

Many backpacking hippies gathered here to enjoy the peace and tranquillity of the sea, sand and laid-back atmosphere. There were Russians, Israelis, Japanese, German, English, and Italian travellers to note and a smattering of other nationalities.

The shack holders didn't have electricity and precariously connected wires to the odd light post wires in order to run a light bulb with risk of electric shock or a fine from the local constabulary. Access was only gained on foot so the locals could see the Police arriving from the distance and act accordingly. hiding any evidence of wrongdoing before problems arose.

To keep the soft drinks cool, Ice Man as we called him, a very strong local amiable fellow carried a massive block of ice from a fish factory several miles away through difficult terrain negotiating cliffs and jungle. This block of ice was over a metre long and 40cm thick and he carried it wrapped in a hemp sack balanced on his head. This strenuous exertion gave him a perfectly developed muscular torso and although almost a thankful task, luckily for him he had the melted water from the ice block to keep him from overheating, carrying this serious weight in the heat of the midday sun.

He was all ready to hail Shiva and deservingly lit up several chillums after his work was done, that is, after he'd mopped his brow and drank a chai. Once he was relaxed and at rest, he would beam and smile, happy his toil was over, his strong white teeth contrasting with his dark, supple skin.

Dolphins, flying fish, jellyfish and other marine life were abundant here in the crystal waters and I had the pleasure of seeing dolphins with their young frolicking in the luminous bright green phosphorescent waters at night squeaking with delight as their bright green torsos played in the brightly lit surf, surely a beauty to behold.

Another night while walking on the moonlit beach, I witnessed a turtle come ashore and lay its eggs, making sure to keep this a secret so that the eggs wouldn't be otherwise poached for an omelette.

Campfires were held at night where various musicians would sit around and jam with guitars, flutes, didgeridoos and drums, passing chillums of charas around to cries of Boom Shiva, Boom Bholenath and Shiva Shambo. I was playing the guitar and knocking out some songs penned by Donovan and Nick Drake. The stars were incredible and many a shooting star was seen, and forgotten, as were the satellites.

The majority of travellers here were constantly baked and blissed out, eating exotic fruits and yoghurt for breakfast, drinking from fresh green coconuts and delicious curries at night. Alcohol was rarely seen, except imbibed by the odd local, as the triad of Chai, Chillum, Chapatti took dominance here.

On Christmas day, a local fisherman took me and a beautiful blonde, buxom English girl called Sarah, who played the mandolin, in his rudimentary sailing boat with ragged, tatty, patched up sails around the headland to the next port of call, Paradise beach where one had to fashion a dwelling for sleep and shade as it was a virgin beach.

I was that baked that I can't remember how

me and the girl communicated, looking back, not being sure if we'd taken strong acid tabs or not in previous days and how our mental states were.

We bowled around topless on the beach, smoking chillums and eating a few onion bhajis and samosas we had brought along, drinking from a fresh water spring, and it would have been an ideal place for making love but I think neither of us were up for it, being way too spaced out.

It tormented me later on in the UK, that I hadn't taken Sarah's contact details when we parted and I longed to see her again, yet to no avail, as our paths never crossed again.

I was to return to Om beach many times over the next five years and funnily enough, the memories all seem to roll into one but this first visit always remained special.

It was time to move on again, and I said goodbye to friends I had made and continued North again, this time to Goa.

12

GOA

With miles upon miles of tropical beaches, winding roads adorned with palm trees, café shacks, tropical fruits and fresh green coconuts, the birthplace of psychedelic trance music and trance parties and a former Portuguese colonial heritage, it's no wonder for decades this exotic destination has been a magnet for hippies and travellers from all over the world.

Goa has Christian links going back as far as Doubting Thomas from the gospel, who is alleged to have travelled and preached here. The Catholic Portuguese settlers were surprised to find a type of Christianity here when they arrived here in the early 16th Century. Throughout the state, you can see white churches reminiscent of what you would expect to find in Mexico.

I hooked up with some other backpacking

adventurers and slept in a hammock in a communal dwelling situated close to the beach. The weather was perfect to bowl around the sleepy villages, where dogs and cows alike lazed in the shade of towering coconut palms. It is truly tropical here with equatorial forests and rich fauna and wildlife.

A young boy wielded a machete with uncomfortable ease to prepare a fresh coconut for me to drink and quench my thirst in the hot sun. First, they chop off the top with the said blade, from which you then drink a delicious refreshing juice with a straw. Then they cleave the husk in two and with a spoon shaped piece of the same coconut shell, you scoop out the inside of the husk, which is like a soft coconut jelly, sweet and white and very tasty indeed.

You could walk to get around or go on one of the many motorbike taxis that would whisk you to your next destination at any time day or night, as you hang on behind the rider being careful not to burn your leg on the exhaust.

Some travellers would buy and travel around on Royal Enfield Motorbikes. Originally built in England, they have been built in India since the 1960s. Designed by the Enfield Cycle Company, the Royal Enfield Bullet is the longest-lived motorcycle design in history. It was popular with Israeli male travellers who were flush with cash after doing their military service in Israel and was the poseur machine to have at this time.

Popular places in Goa included Anjuna beach and its flea market, Arambol, Israeli Beach, Spaghetti Beach, The Primrose Café, Fort Aguada, Vagator Beach and Hilltop.

At Anjuna flea market, having broken sandals, I came across some bejewelled brightly dressed tribal women from Karnataka who offered to make me some suitable footwear. The soles they used were fashioned from discarded car tyres and the upper material from intricate hand-woven colourful material embedded with circular mirrors and delicately stitched patterns, a typical trademark of these Karnatakan tribes people. Having paid over the odds but happy with the result, they looked like a medieval footwear one would see Asterix wearing but on an acid trip, such were the vibrant colours. These shoes were unique and comfortable, strong yet crazy which apparently suited my mood.

Here you would say well-worn aged hippies who had arrived in the sixties and seemingly never left. They would sell hippy garments, chillums and other Asian artefacts and often make a living travelling around Asia buying and selling, sometimes returning to Europe in the summertime to sell at festivals.

On the white beaches, the sun seekers would catch rays, smoke chillums and play chess, backgammon and the Indian Carrom board in the chai shacks and cafes dotted along the sands while listening to music. Carrom board, like a miniature pool table, is played on a square board with counters, which have to be flicked against one another to pot them in the pockets at the corner. It's highly entertaining and addictive and requires a high degree of skill and dexterity to become a master player.

Travellers and Indians alike would while away the hours chilling in such pursuits or relaxing in hammocks when things got too heavy man, sipping on a freshly squeezed strawberry juice to cool down. Shanti Shanti

Goa trance parties would occur on every full moon and other auspicious dates as well throughout the relatively short season between November and February, outside these months the overwhelming heat and humidity becomes a problem, being hot and sticky. Travellers would usually then head slowly north to the mountains via Rajasthan, Madhya Pradesh and Omkareshwar in pursuit of cooler climes and fresh air ready for the next charas harvest in early autumn.

These tribal trance gatherings would occur at Disco Valley, Hill Top, The Primrose Café and Bamboo Forest bringing together an eclectic mix of world travellers who wanted to dance and trance away the night in spectacular settings to the latest underground Goan Trance music that the old school hippies had created. Minidisc was a popular format for the DJs as the sound quality was excellent, and being so small, easily to transport around.

Local Goan women would spread out blankets and set up temporary chai shops to sell to the party goers who would be in varying degrees of (in)sanity and inebriation. Chillums would be flared up and passed around during the night until and after sunrise as the music carried on pulsating through the generator powered sound systems. Trance music has a recurring repetitive beat interspersed with sound effects or samples and mixed with melodies making the dancer feel at one with the Universe, euphoric, ecstatic and mystic.

Acid drops and LSD tabs would be openly available and the energy under these palm or bamboo surrounded dance floors was electric. The dance floor was just dry earth, a stone's throw from the beach, with luminescent paintings and the jenny lamps of the chai vendors providing light alongside of course the full moon beams shining through the palm trees.

Hearing about these parties was by word of mouth and I somehow managed to come across several of these by apparent accident or chance.

A famous old-school DJ who still continues to spin the wheels of steel around the globe is Goa Gil and I had the pleasure to be at several of his parties around the Christmas of 1995.

Dance. Dance is active meditation. When we dance, we go beyond thought, beyond mind and beyond our own individuality, to become one in the divine ecstasy of the union with the cosmic spirit. This is the essence of the trance dance experience. Hare Hare Mahadev, Om Namah Shivaya. Goa Gil-

After such hedonism, I decided to head back to Karnataka but this time inland to the Ancient temples and UNESCO heritage sight of Hampi.

13

HAMPI

After a bumpy, dusty bus journey, I arrived at this destination, which seemed like a land forgotten. Bullocks hauled hay carts down the main dusty concourse and grubby restaurants offered delicious snacks and southern food such as masala dosas and idli.

The Hindu text Ramayana dates back to around 7323BC and many scholars believe the places described in this epic bear close resemblances to the geography found at Hampi, and therefore attracting pilgrims. It was the world's second-largest medieval city after Beijing in 1500AD, attracting traders from Persia and Portugal. The Vijayanagara Empire was defeated by a coalition of Muslim sultanates; its capital was conquered, pillaged and destroyed by Sultanate armies in 1565, after which Hampi remained in ruins.

To reach the temples, which are scattered over a 16 square mile site, one has to leave the new main town centre and cross the river. Ferryman shift passengers across this river famed for dangerous currents, eddies and whirlpools.

The boats, remarkably, are coracles, round basket shaped hulls formed from branches, animal hides and coated in tar to increase impermeability. It didn't sail, but span to the other side with the ferryman paddling with strength, experience and skill to avoid mishap.

Off I stepped, bag on one shoulder and blanket on the other, in my fashioned Asterix boots into another world in the middle of southern India.

Great orange and pink granite rock formations dominated the landscape, which was undulating and hilly, contrasted by a mix of lush green vegetation and arid dust.

Between these rocks were the Ancient Temples, pillars and buildings of grandeur days now long since gone by and amongst these manmade and natural stone structures lived Tribal people of a Dravidian nature in colourful garments that grew rice and harvested opium.

The sun beat down relentlessly from a crystal blue sky as I wandered through this foreign landscape taking it all in.

I found refuge in a straw roofed mud hut thrown up by locals to take advantage of the tourist trade and stayed here for a few weeks investigating the surrounding area, sketching and taking photos. I met up with a beautiful German girl and an English fellow with whom I smoked Opium sourced from the locals.

To this day I don't know if I smoked it for six days solid, as I lost total track of time and any sense of reality, or in fact it was six weeks. If you've ever tried this narcotic, I can say it tasted almost Chinese in flavour, powerful and addictive leaving me on a different planet, not knowing if I was capable of talking or acting coherently.

High on this drug of the east, I shambled on to a village where a bizarre spectacle was taking place. A group of villagers, outside their medieval, rustic, thatched, one-room dwellings, were gathered round an oil drum with a blazing fire burning inside whilst one of the villagers dressed in lunghi and sandals lifted a cobra in a pair of tongues and dropped it into the flames.

I thought I was witnessing some crazy sacrifice to one of the pantheon of the gods but I discovered later that it had a very practical explanation. The cobra had been discovered in one of the huts and killed, and to prevent its mate from following its scent and exacting its revenge on the warpath on the death of its mate, it was burnt to remove any trace or evidence.

A couple I'd met on the beach in Gokarna also came to Hampi, Gaz and Jane from Blackpool. Friendly folk, Gaz worked on the Pleasure Beach during the summer and travelled in winters to more idyllic locations than his hometown. He liked his LSD but his trip went awry while in Hampi, he'd taken a strong one and it was really torqueing his mind.

He was marching round the boulders and

rocks amid dust and vegetation clasping and gesturing into thin air, dreadlocks flying, dressed in psychedelic apparel and sandals and brandishing a staff convinced he was Jesus or God or maybe both. For the observer it was amusing, and we just puffed on chillums and laughed till his high wore off. For Gaz it was a living hell of confusion, contorting his brain and soul trying to make some sense of it all, this temporary insanity, not unlike bad trips I'd experienced. For some people it's a one-way ticket from which they never recover or return to normality, however you choose to define it, or the illusion of such.

Another day I made my way to the Monkey Temple perched on a high outcrop of rock giving way to splendid views of this tropical colourful epic site with rivers, rocks and ancient monuments. Here lived a sadhu, not alone, but with monkeys who are represented by Hanuman in Hindu scripture. The Rhesus Macaque are Asian Old-World monkeys and are the most popular primate to be found in India and I never grew tired of watching their comical behaviour and antics, for the most part, enjoying their company and displays more than with fellow human beings. Dogs bring me similar joy with their uncomplicated way of being and existing but these monkeys even more so, with their displays at times identical to human behaviour.

I smoked a few chillums with the sadhu while he conversed with some Indian tourist pilgrims and the monkeys had free reign of the place.

Later on I found an inviting lagoon in which to have a dip but quickly changed my mind after seeing a snake (I think it was a king cobra complete with a large hood) arise from the water with a fish in its fangs.

Hampi was a dreamy place, somehow unspoilt and mystic, ancient and spiritual, vibrant and colourful. Energy seemed to pulsate from the land itself and the huge granite boulders, changed their hues depending on the sun, as did the sky with scorching red sunsets fusing into purple, blue and black.

It was time to move on, leaving this surreal landscape to exist for many more millennia, and I headed east to Hyderabad.

As I crossed the border into Andra Pradesh, the bus I was bouncing along on was stopped, and the bus duly boarded by Police. Being a 'dry state' where alcohol was prohibited, they were looking for anyone contravening the rules and smuggling in a bit of tipple. Being the only white face on the bus, I was immediately singled out and asked for my bag to be searched. I wasn't carrying any alcohol but had a stash of charas which would have caused problems if found. I did what I amusingly refer to as a Jedi mind trick. Having two bags, I simply gave them the bag with no incriminating products inside which they ransacked to no avail and after examining my passport, disappointedly concurred all was in order and let the bus proceed to the capital. Breathing a sigh of relief, I chuckled to the devout Muslim beside me who was wearing a prayer cap, "the booze is in the other bag" to which he gave me a shocked, dirty look. Allahu Akbar!

I stayed at a distant friends of my father's, an Irish nurse who had married an Indian doctor while working in the UK and had since retired to his native place. I think they were shocked by my ragged hippy appearance and carryings on but were very hospitable and welcoming and had a driver shuttle me about to see the sights and a cook who provided amazing food.

My trip was coming to an end, as was my one-year visa, so I soon boarded a train to New Delhi where I was scheduled to meet my brother for the last ten days of my stay in India.

So I finally boarded an Uzbekistani aeroplane once more, stopping in miserable Tashkent airport which was some kind of Communist barn of a place where one could only buy feck all in dollars. Fat, shot-putting women boarded the plane with hens in a cage and took no shit from anyone and pushed and shoved to the best seats. Funnily enough, you could smoke on the back three rows of the plane, making this shuddering dodgy airplane feel more like a bus to Butlin's.

During my Indian trip, I'd had a recurring nightmare that I'd returned to the UK and was then trapped and couldn't get back to my ventures in India. How true this nightmare was going to turn out was uncanny, but as the whole year in India had been one long stoned adventure, I didn't really realise what I was in for once I hit UK soil.

I was totally unaware and unprepared for the culture

shock on my return. I'd settled into a carefree existence, only contemplating my next chillum, next meal or next trip within India, going with the flow and seemingly always surrounded by positive happy, friendly helpful people.

14

GRIM UP NORTH

Back at my parent's house, after my belongings had been searched at the airport by custom's officials at Manchester airport, I was, alas, instantly lost. Everything was cold and sterile and revolved around the television. The streets were empty and everyone drove round in cars, seemingly in a desperate rush to get nowhere. Only dead legs, pensioners and school kids travelled by public transport and everyone kept themselves to themselves. Alone, I sought the companionship of old friends who were busy working and had little time to meet up.

When I did eventually meet friends, it was in a pub and they got shitfaced within two hours and the depth of conversation disappeared. At a loss, I too followed suit and began to drink after a year's break: the consequences came rapid and hard.

Living with my parents was impossible and

suffocating, with constant remarks like, 'You need to find a job,' and 'What are you going to do?' – totally alien concepts to me at the time, as my heart and soul and one foot were still in India, and my mind was becoming ever more fragile, bombarded with drab television soaps, graphic news images of wars and conflicts, and the main concern seemingly the division one football match between whoever.

I quickly agreed to rent a room in a friend's house, where I slept on pallets with a sleeping bag and spent most of the day looking at photos I'd taken in India, wishing I was back there and regretting ever coming back. In fact, such was the impact of missing India, I began trying to pretend I *was* in India to make me feel better, which is something I still do twenty-something years later on.

I'd put on some Hindi Bollywood cassettes on the stereo, sit cross legged on my blanket which I'd decorated and embroidered whilst in India, and it had become my talisman. I'd smoke whatever cannabis Indica or Sativa, hash or grass I could get my hands on and eat curry and drink chai.

But however hard I tried, it made me miss India even more and I was totally a fish out of water. Spending most days alone, at odds with the rat race and everyone else's busy nine to five routine, I started to drink heavily, with or without friends, wandering the streets and moors, parks and hills, trying to seek solace in nature, but it was early spring and the weather was cold and rough. The vibe was totally at odds with what I had become accustomed to in the shanti, laid back peaceful Indian countryside. A northern town can be edgy, aggressive and unforgiving to the sensitive soul. Coupled with this was my insufficient lack of funds to fund my smoking habit and drinking, and the vice began to tighten both emotionally and financially until something gave way.

Soon my mind had regressed to the fragile state it had been in pre-India and I was not in a good way. having delusional thoughts and paranoias. I was out of control.

My parents took me to a GP and from there I was admitted to a psychiatric institution – a secure unit, also known as heartbreak hotel, the madhouse or funny farm. I was totally broken and my marvellous Indian adventure, now just a dream and a lifetime away. I'd lost everything in a matter of weeks; my mind, my freedom, my pride, my will to live, my ability to be normal and my independence.

If there was rock bottom, this was it, as I slept in a ward with other cases, was given medication, monitored, questioned and supervised by the hospital staff. Although a secure unit, I did manage to escape for the sheer hell of it, to prove to myself that I could. I was completely bored, dwindling away the hours chain-smoking my fingers brown waiting for a meal, or a visit or to go to bed and sleep, which I found was the only time I wasn't depressed.

Once I had escaped, I felt better, and calmly walked back to Hillside as it was named. You would get all sorts in these mental institutions, old and young, male and female, withdrawn and aggressive, funny and scary…and that was just the nurses!

One of the other patients in the unit, was an ex-policeman and we chatted about God-knows-what as we smoked. Bit by bit, we were allowed out to explore the hospital grounds and go for walks, and I saw him one day heading down the road so I decided to follow him from a safe distance, just out of curiosity to see where he was going. The things you do when you have feck all to do. Eventually after a few miles, he'd clocked me so I dived down an alley out of sight,

That evening, back in the unit, he was perplexed, angry and confused why I'd been following him to which I had no obvious answer but I thought; 'You're the copper, you work it out', and found it hilarious that I'd been following a policeman instead of the other way round.

Apparently after a while my condition slightly improved and I was moved to a less secure hospital wing where if my condition improved I would be allowed weekend releases.

So, time went by with the hospital meals, the psychiatrist's report and weekly interviews, therapeutic workshops, cocoa before bed and medication time. I'd seen Jack Nicholson in *One Flew Over the Cuckoo's Nest*, but although we didn't have Red Indians on the ward chewing Juicy Fruit, we had the odd Pakistani.

One day, I became angry as my dad had my credit card and I was planning to catch a train to Birmingham and do one from this hellish place, but without money it was impossible.

I attempted to storm out of the ward but the door was locked as it had gone closing time, so I just kicked the reinforced glass out of the door and broke out.

A happier moment was during the summer and the World Cup was on in which I had absolutely no interest and I came in from the garden with my ghetto blaster on my shoulder, walking through the ward blaring out Bob Marley. Unfortunately, that too got smashed up in a fit of rage.

Every patient had their own story to tell on the ward, if you could be bothered listening. There was the teenage skinhead with "possessed" crudely tattooed on his arm who would steal anything, having been raised in childcare facilities all his life and was now in some Bible bashing, born again Christian cult, and I couldn't stand him.

Then there was a likeable lad who liked his rock n roll and blues but would come crying back to the ward having yet again taken amphetamines. This would leave him in a right state, a weeping quivering wreck, vowing never to touch the drug again.

There was a red headed ex-football hooligan who after many years of being some kind of hard man, was now a pathetic, sad excuse of a man and a coward.

An ex-squaddie was in a similar boat but had a bit more about him as he'd travelled with his job.

There was an eccentric, wild, ginger-haired, bearded mathematics genius who had cracked under the pressure of one too many formulae or theories, that slept in the bed next to mine. He was very quiet and kept himself to himself but snored like a train. He had a vase of flowers by his bedside which his mother had brought him but, genius or not, his snoring got the better of me and the vase of water over his head soon put a stop to that. He awoke with a fright, all wet and I assured him "it's raining."

There was a very old man, over six-foot-tall who smoked a pipe and enthused about his time on the continent. He was a connoisseur of fine Dutch tobaccos and knew his different shags and flavours. We had an interesting conversation about this one evening in the smoking TV lounge (or he spoke and I listened). The next night, he told the very same story, almost word for word, and the night after that and on the fourth night I avoided conversing with him. He was afflicted with memory loss or some kind of dementia or Alzheimer's, poor chap.

They'd tried different medications on the pipe smoker to no avail, so they tried electrotherapy on him one day: the cold, sharp shock treatment. You'd always know when someone had had it done as they'd wheel them back in on a stretcher to their room and the nurses pretended nothing had happened, not unlike *Cuckoo's Nest*. That night – I'll never forget it – I had a dream of the grim reaper by my bedside, a dream I've never had before or again.

In the morning, as the patients were having breakfast, the hospital porters were only wheeling out the pipe smoker, dead as a dodo, under a blanket (less than 24 hours after having the electrotherapy) to the morgue to rest on a cold slab. Game over, buddy.

Now, for a patient to get the electro shock therapy (which has always seemed to me to be barbaric, without scientific reasoning or justification) someone in your family has to sign authorisation papers for you to undergo this medieval ritual if your psychiatrist has suggested it as a solution.

I'd met a lad, a year younger than me, in the

next ward who had happened to go to the same school as I had and was a child prodigy. He'd excelled at Maths, sports, literature and was a great artist and had been the greatest achiever in his year, head and shoulders above the rest. On top of this, he had never succumbed to the evils of drugs or drink and was a fairly quiet boy, possibly overprotected and pushed academically by his parents.

I visited him a few times and we played chess, which I assume he won every time. Anyway, he wasn't responding to conventional medication and his parents were offered electrotherapy. Obviously desperate to regain the successful boy they had once had, they agreed to the shock treatment. I heard, years later, that he'd never left home, he continued to live with his parents, a shadow of the prodigy he had once been, shuffling around in his slippers, possibly what is harshly known on the street as 'a cabbage'.

So I count myself lucky I never had the shock treatment and maybe once the drugs and alcohol were out of my system my brain slowly started to function again and piece itself back together. I must note that there was a history of psychiatric problems running back in my family line to my grandfather. Whether the drugs had triggered or exacerbated this genetic default, begs a question.

15

DIAGNOSIS

Came the day when my psychiatrist gave me his diagnosis: schizophrenia.

I'm not sure if I'd been aware of the term before, but when he said it to me, it was like a knife tearing me apart, destroying my previously colourful, happy, naïve soul.

I totally broke down in uncontrollable tears and raged at the apparent harshness of the sentence and the sheer brutality of what he was saying, looking for some way out, in denial, cornered and totally trapped, alone and completely broken and useless.

I struggled with the diagnosis for a long time, like a wild, rabid wolf in a cage, thinking it had to be a mistake: a conspiracy to cut my wings, to punish me for smoking an illegal substance, for trying to be different and go head-on against the status quo. I wrestled with the term schizophrenia until I was so depressed, down and broken, I had no choice but to meekly accept it, take the medicine and join the queue with the other losers and plebs and toe the line. I'd thrived on an alternative path, challenging the status quo of governments and warmongering, always concerned about the state of the environment, rejecting capitalism and multinationals and tuning in and dropping out of the conventional rat-race, but now I paid a heavy price. Madness, insanity and none of the flower children or happy-go-lucky hippies were here to help me in my hour of need.

I guess it's what you could call a serious reality check and, although years later I'm still a fairly free spirit, I believe I've seen both sides of the coin, giving me a unique viewpoint that not all in this world is as it seems. I know people who have escaped the trials of mental institutions and carried on regardless, not needing such help or support, but I feel it has eventually made me stronger, definitely a more complex and complicated individual who sees things sometimes in a completely different light to most people. Yes, I've travelled to the dark side and come back and not many can truly claim that.

I've experienced euphoria and torment, yet still have faith in the mystic and omnipotent powers that be, and happily seek truth in world religions and cultures, be it Hinduism, Buddhism, Christianity, Rastafari, pagan worship, the Sky Gods of the Mughals, the Mother Earth of Native Americans and the oneness of everything. Devotion to your path can lead to fulfilling your destiny and making you feel a part of this crazy, wonderful brotherhood. To be in harmony with nature has to be a goal if we have any form of self-respect, intelligence or wisdom.

Rich people (in the monetary sense) might be clever, but that is not to say they are wise – alas the state of the Planet is driven by greed and wealth, and deemed successful by the majority.

Bob Marley was once interviewed by Australian reporter, George Negus:

Negus:	Are you a rich man?
Bob:	What you mean rich, what ya mean?
Negus:	Do you have a lot of possessions? Lot of money in the bank?
Bob:	Possession make you rich? I don't have that type of richness. My richness is life, forever.

I have made many mistakes, and that is how one learns, never underestimate the perils and dangers of choosing the less trodden path. Following everybody else can give an easier, comfortable and less complicated life, even though those you are following are sheep or lemmings or the proverbial lamb to the slaughter.

"It's better to have tried and failed than to live life wondering what would've happened if I tried."

Alfred, Lord Tennyson

After four months, I was free to go: on the condition I took medication (Amisulpride) daily for the rest of my life, which was a bitter pill to swallow.

After the highs of insanity came chronic depression, which would hang over me like a ghost, unable to shake it off. Wishing I was in India, wishing I was dead, suicidal thoughts, black thoughts and confusion with no obvious way out.

I'd tried smoking hash to escape this living nightmare but it left me more depressed and confused than ever, forcing me into bed under the duvet, hoping the mental torture would end.

The advice from the psychiatrist was that I could "have a drink but don't get drunk". Work that one out!

I went without alcohol and marijuana for a year, socialising with ginger beer, fruit juice, lemonade or the terrible alcohol-free beer, Kaliber. Socialising was difficult when all my friends were getting drunk, and it's quite a bizarre thing being a nightclub and being the only one sober. It was so boring, but better than staring at the four walls and nice to see my friends.

Constantly going through my mind was how things had been so different in India, free as a bird, without a care in the world. In fact, life before had been plain sailing during my youth and university days, completing my studying and leaving ample time for playing football with friends, socialising and living it up at bars and parties.

I was tormented by the fact that I couldn't bliss out and smoke a joint as before, relaxing my mood and feeing great. I felt like the character Obelix who had fallen into the magic potion and was always annoyed he couldn't partake in the elixir like everyone else in the village. Everywhere I looked I saw the influences of drugs and alcohol and felt it unfair that I had been cruelly ejected from this sub-culture. On the radio, songs with drug references and artists clearly under the influence, advertisements using Jimi Hendrix music and psychedelic imagery, and other friends imbibing as never before without a hint of negative or problematic repercussions, rugby or football matches with alcoholic sponsorship, pubs on every corner and supermarkets seemingly giving it away. All these things served to torment me and leave me in anguish.

I couldn't get moving or create any momentum being so down and was waiting for nothing to happen; melancholic about the past, despondent in the present and couldn't see any positivity coming from the future.

I started to go to jam nights in an attempt to socialise more, lift my spirits and give me a focus, playing the odd song on guitar and singing the occasional tune I'd written. It was a release and got me mixing with new people and, for a while, I'd come out of myself and enjoyed a few hours away from the confines of the flat.

I guess that's why they call it the blues.

I was still obsessed with India and not a day went by when I didn't wish I could smoke cannabis again, confused by what I read in mental health reviews and media: that it was only psychologically addictive and easy to stop. To this day I don't know what 'psychologically addictive' means, and it sounds like horseshit to me: some people find it easier to stop than others.

I'd tried a few times miserably to enjoy a puff or two but this again put me in a bad way, running for the duvet. I drove my mental health nurse crazy because it's all I talked about and after months of talking with me, exasperated with my plight, she suggested I tried smoking it again, being at her wits end with me. I pleaded with her that I needed it to function. Period.

On the suggestion of my parents, I applied to work as a volunteer in a Christian centre in Hertfordshire and was duly accepted. I spent maybe six or nine months there, and the people were friendly and looked after me well. They were possibly all devout Catholics, but my faith in anything had been killed by depression, and I found no spiritual solace in stale Christian teachings. I just zombied my way through, heavily medicated, always tired, always depressed. But looking back, it was the social interaction I needed, to help me pick up the broken pieces of my life and grow stronger and regain my confidence. The religious atmosphere I found stifling but there was good camaraderie between the volunteers and they accepted me for who I was, flaws and all.

Finally, after time spent there sober, I felt strong enough to move on somewhere else and I'd saved a bit of money. There was little to spend my allowance on except cigarettes and alcohol and I wasn't drinking at this stage.

I met a girl at a festival there and was besotted with her. We had a bit of a fling, but my heart was set on going to India and I hoped to see her on my return.

When this volunteer sabbatical ended, I returned to Manchester and after completing a year alcohol and drug free, I tried again, smoking a very light joint and it wasn't so bad. I felt an elevated high, disconnected from reality for a while. I lit an incense stick, put on some psychedelic trance and shed the shackles and weight I'd been carrying arduously for so long. I'd been taking the anti-depressant Prozac for months, which may have lifted my spirits, but the effects were negligible and carried side effects so I happily exchanged these chemicals for my regular fix of THC. Slowly, I could start rolling, literally, a bit of rock n roll in my life again propelling me into more creative and diverse avenues and directions, my confidence and self-belief slowly returning and I could only now start planning a little bit ahead having regained the optimism to carry me.

I visited friends in old haunts in Birmingham and London, travelling by train, taking up where I'd left off before going the Indian subcontinent, living as a rolling stone.

I busked on the tube in London and headed down to Brixton looking to score some weed, asking some winos outside the tube station where I could find some gear. One man, stinking of alcohol, with a can of Tennent's Super in his hand and a fag in the other, looked at me and said "Don't go asking anyone, man, I could be a copper for all you know". He continued to give me directions to Tony the Dealer, a few miles away.

I finally found his house on a council estate in a rough area and was chancing it but nonetheless he let me into his chaotic bungalow. His wife had cerebral palsy or some kind of paralysis and was wheelchair bound and the house was in a right state, with bare floors and two long haired German shepherds sleeping off the smoky haze and the odd cat here and there. Their young son was half wild but cute and likeable with it and was always up to some mischief or other, a true rogue, with Tony bawling at him to "Stop that! Do this!" or "Behave!" as he carried on regardless.

Tony's was going to be my port of call whenever I was in London for the next few years. He weighed out grass or hash on the old type scales, making sure to boil it over a boiling pan of water in a sieve which he said freshened the taste but what he was in fact doing was adding artificial weight to the deal so you ended up getting less for your money. Being relieved to be stoned anyway, you didn't realise or care what was going on as long as you got out of there as quickly and cheaply as possible. He'd fleece you, but was no threat, and commented that he had many sad cases such as myself teetering on the verge of mental instability and the smoke kept us quiet and ticking over. As it happened, the Bush Doctor, Tony, had come over from India in his late teens and had never returned, having worked on the railways in London for many years. He enjoyed telling the story that when he first arrived on the plane to England, he brought with him a bag of ganja seeds to plant, totally unaware it was illegal.

In Birmingham, I had friends who were good to me and put me up for days at a time while they worked and I bummed about. They cooked lovely food for me and we had some great nights out at reggae venues in Moseley and wonderful kushi houses offering up great cheap cuisine cooked up by Birmingham's thriving Asian community. Birmingham always seemed less edgy than Manchester with a more diverse alternative scene and a more inclusive mix and harmony between the various communities, be they Caribbean, Asian or Irish, possibly helped by the large influx of students at the polytechnics and universities.

I had a charas connection here from Mick, who made trips down to a friend in London to get the Indian gear, but hash and weed was freely available with the local Rastafari community providing a good service. Looking back, I regretted ever returning to Manchester after India, as it was Birmingham I had been living in for close on five years before my journey. I felt at home there, more accepted and relaxed than I did in Manchester.

Smoking wasn't without its hiccups though and I had to be careful not to overdo it, being easily susceptible to paranoia, although none of the fanatical delusions I'd suffered from previously.

What I had to cope with now is what the medical profession would call "hearing voices". To the layman, it's like random voices or ideas that pop into your head that may be delusional, bizarre, frightening, macabre, amusing, vulgar or in fact can take any form. It's as if you're in a dream state but awake, not fully in control of your mind. These can be brought on through high amounts of stress or damage to the brain through abuse of toxicants such as I had experienced. Let's not forget, many cases of nervous breakdowns and psychotic episodes can happen without the use or abuse of narcotics or alcohol, triggered by a genetic defect or some kind of psychological shock such as the loss of a loved one, a marriage breakup or being exposed to trauma or extreme violence. It can be compared to a shutting down of the cerebral functions; the brain and soul saying it's had enough and can't take anymore.

Literature circling mental hospitals mentions Biblical figures experiencing hearing voices, like Moses, but I didn't find this too helpful – I needed to steer away from the idea I was driven by some mystical force, in an attempt to regain my own sanity.

Coping strategies for hearing voices suggested by care workers and doctors alike proved useful in an attempt to ignore the voices, but there's a fine line between a normal idea projected by the brain and a delusional thought. Differentiating between these different thought processes occurring in one's consciousness can mean the difference between success and failure, and as one progresses and hopefully improves one's mental stability, it is vital to cut out the chaff from the wheat.

A good quote that comes to mind is:

"There is a fine line between genius and madness. I have erased this line."

The multifaceted genius, Oscar Levant

Apparently, recent medical reports have found conclusive links between creativity and mental illnesses such as schizophrenia.

Scientists have discovered that creative people

have a gene called neuregulin 1 in common, which is also linked to psychosis and depression. In fact, it plays a role in brain development but a variant of it is linked to mental illnesses like schizophrenia and bipolar disorder (Semmelweis University, Hungary).

So I slowly reverted into a similar lifestyle I'd had before my breakdown, although with less energy and in fear of a repeat of being committed to another psychiatric ward. I slept a lot and wasn't as impulsive as before and avoided reckless risk taking and hard drug taking. I smoked mainly roll ups and cannabis and drank alcohol occasionally as it interfered with my medicine, wiping me out so that I'd need 12 hours to sleep it off. I became more serious, less adventurous and developed a grumpier, more irritable trait to my personality, brought on by constant tiredness, a side effect of the medication and frustration with my situation. Maybe it was an unwilling first step into maturing somewhat, from a happy naïve youth to a more serious adult. I probably never wanted to grow up or accept the responsibility an adult life brings as I was never happier than when in my youth. Intoxicants had stalled and initially eased this process, putting pressures on pause for a while, but yes, getting older was unfortunately inevitable and I'd eventually complicated my life becoming addicted to such vices.

I wanted to be back in India and wished I'd never been in hospital, but I was stuck here in an old town outside Manchester with no job and no prospects of one considering my unwillingness, inability and lack of desire to work. Something had died in me, a part of my creative spirit, my enthusiasm for life, my happy go lucky nature, my constant smile and I wanted it back. The only way I thought this could be achieved was by returning to India and picking up the pieces of my broken heart and soul. In doing so, I was hoping to forget this traumatic stage of my life, put it behind me and move on, hopefully picking up the energy and momentum I'd had previously. Pure escapism, but this showed my spirit was still fighting and just about flickering, despite being fragile and broken.

I did a bit of volunteer work to get me back into society, delivering meals on wheels to pensioners in the village and the odd gardening job. I helped out at the local church and ran errands and did odd jobs for my parents, but I was just biding my time until I could get a flight back to India.

16

RETURN TO INDIA

I don't know or remember how, but somehow, I organised another flight to India, putting together cash from here and there. India had become an obsession, not going one day without the thought of it luring me back, like I was under a spell. I've met many similar travellers to India who have never left the place, such is its power and the hold it can have on people, and I too was in its grip. I'm not exactly sure why this happens, but when you let the culture, people and places of India under your skin, there's nothing like it and you want more and more, like an on-going love affair. The reality in India is a different reality to the one found in the UK and the rollercoaster ride of emotions one experiences in vast Hindustan leaves one in awe, constantly surprised, delighted and shocked. It's a vibrant, wild and crazy place, beautiful, sometimes terrible but never dull or boring.

As soon as the warm air hit me as I disembarked the plane steps in New Delhi, my body tingled and a sense of joy and homecoming overwhelmed me and I knew this is where I wanted to be right here, right now. At my lowest depressed points since hospital, I'd doubted at times actually ever being here, dismissing it as an impossible dream, not believing such happiness had existed, but here I was, going for it again.

I knew my way around this time and wanted to revisit old haunts during this six-month visit, the legendary one-year visa had now been discontinued.

I stayed again on Om beach, being only one of three travellers as I was there before the season had started and we delighted in this unspoilt paradise. We tried to seek shade and made do with simple food, smoking chillums all day long, keeping an eye out for the weary policeman who would patrol the beach and be sweating profusely on arrival due to walking miles from the local town to reach us in his uniform in the intense heat.

We moved to Paradise beach for a few weeks and took it in turns to bring supplies from Gokarna, often returning alone at night negotiating jungle, rocks and cliffs with or without a rudimentary torch.

The beaches hadn't lost their charm, the golden sand, the crystal waters and lush tropical vegetation. Interesting travellers from around the world trickled in as the season got under way and there was a great vibe to the place.

A side effect of my tablets for schizophrenia was that they inhibit the pigmentation process in the skin that allows it to go brown and form a suntan. So there I was, three months on a tropical beach and glowing white as a sheet as other travellers topped up their tans, that's life.

I think it was here, totally blissed out, that I decided I was fine without my medication and stopped taking it. Bholenath.

Again, I seemed fine in India, having stopped drinking alcohol and enjoying the stress-free existence, but only time would tell. I didn't really grasp the gravity of what I was doing at the time, totally unaware and stoned.

I revisited beautiful Hampi and returned to Goa for the inevitable trance parties and returned to the Himalaya, spending time with my father in Dharamshala and Naggar, Kullu valley, Himachal Pradesh. It was all as I had left it, and it lived up to my expectations once again.

But all good things come to an end and it was time to return to England. I thought I might try living in London on my return, God knows why.

I'd been talked into bringing back some charas with me and was given the hash on credit, having to pay the next time I returned to India. Swallowing large capsules of charas at four in the morning isn't easy or advisable when you're stoned and half asleep before getting ready to fly to London, but that's what I was doing and I'd got a new T-shirt to look presentable at customs.

My friend who picked me up in London wasn't well amused as, apparently, I had head lice and then came the grim task of ejecting the charas from my digestive system. A messy job.

Anyway, it kept me in smokes for a while and I rented a room in a flat with some students in Tooting Bec. But again, I was a fish out of water, all alone in a city of 10 million, couldn't get enough to smoke, driven mad by the hassles of the busy city and I foolishly started drinking again. I'd obviously not worked out that I was following exactly the same path I'd taken before which had lead me into the psychiatric hospital in the first place.

The fast pace of life a metropolis such as London has and the large amount of money needed just to survive made my stay here untenable and unsustainable. There are always bars and clubs open and I was ricocheting around boozers and the like, like a silver ball in a pinball machine.

I'd wake up and hit the streets, jumping the tube and sometimes getting caught and carried my chequebook to pay whenever necessary. I sold "Ich tolla" 10 grams of Charas to my old Uni friend, Sean who'd studied at Eton and was now drifting from reggae into Buddhism. We'd seen Lenny Kravitz perform in Birmingham years earlier but had taken such a concoction of drugs before the concert I couldn't speak. The warm-up act, Blind Melon came on and the music was electric, the lead singer Shannon Hoon subsequently died soon after in 1995 from a cocaine overdose while I was in India.

Sean would later get involved in a worrying cult called Universal Medicine, masterminded by the fraud, Serge

Benhayon, and to this day is still brainwashed and trapped there. I'm not sure if his wife and two daughters are involved too which is worrying, I don't know why the authorities can't do anything. The Law is an Ass.

Anyway, back to The Smoke and I was going through copious amounts of charas, hash and marijuana. One night I was somewhere in London and had ran out. I bumped into a second generation West Indian guy who said he'd sort me out. We went to a taxi rank and through a small door leading upstairs, which was a secret kind of speak easy with a bar where we got some drinks and smoked some of his weed. Money changed hands and I got my sunshine in a bag, but we hooked up then for most of the night. I was being taken for a ride but wasn't compos mentis and everything seemed fine at the time. We left there – me with a bottle of Holsten Pils – and next thing we were driving over London Bridge in a Ford Granada saloon taxi with the music pumping and the lights of London shining, smoking and drinking in the back like I'd just won the pools. We frequented a few more establishments and I cashed a few cheques in a Bureau de Change as we partied away the night, finally going back to my flat. Little did I realise at the time, but my new found acquaintance was a crack head or into some other similar Class A hard drug and was covertly putting rocks into our joints which had blown my socks off, already being in a delicate state to start off with. I remember that this hustler was calling chat-lines or something similar on the flat landline in my oblivious state, as we continued to indulge in intoxicants until everything was finished.

We took another taxi to score some more gear, and he left me waiting in the taxi as he took my money to do the deal in a block of flats. He didn't return with drugs or the money and realising I'd been fleeced, returned home, paying the taxi driver by cheque and crashed out.

So I'd exacerbated my already fragile mental state by smoking crack, or coke, or whatever that white rock was, all night, mixed with a lot of alcohol and it was truly a downward spiral.

The following Monday was bleak and, out of money, I convinced an Irish shop keeper to sell me some filterless Player's Navy Cut cigarettes, paying by cheque.

A couple of days later, obviously not right in the head or recovered from smoking crack, I perused the charity shops in Wood Green and got myself a Giorgio Armani American style college jacket and found an Irish pub offering a pitcher of Foster's and bacon and cabbage for £5. Not used to drinking lager and it was the middle of the day, I ate the meal and polished off four pints of Foster's and was staggering around the pub, offending and upsetting people and eventually got thrown out. Enraged by my apparently unfair treatment I stumbled round and finally calmed down in a park and smoked away. I'd asked a policeman for the address of a girl I'd met when I was at the Christian centre and found her address but just waited outside the block of flats hoping on a chance meeting. Night-time came and I eventually bedded down on some old mattresses that had been thrown out.

I awoke early morning and went to the toilet

in the park and then came across a futuristic building, which I think happened to be the local law courts. My mind was flying and again I was on some crazy mission, totally confused so I decided to take a closer look at the building. As I entered there was a security guard and a screening device and I just bolted through it and carried on running with the security guard in hot pursuit. I went down a maze of corridors and through rooms and doors, through the kitchens and jumped out of a fire exit door into a rear car park and just kept on running, waving at another security guard on the parking booth as I left.

I wandered the streets walking miles, going through housing estates, passing Tottenham Hotspurs' football ground, along White hart lane and eventually made it into Tottenham Hale train station at about four in the afternoon and it was dark already. I jumped onto the tracks and climbed up the other side and a rail worker came out, shouting at me across the platform. He appeared aggressive and I deludedly thought he'd said he was going to cut me up. I went completely mad and ripped off my shirt and jacket, socks and trainers, going into some Kung Fu workout alone on the platform, wearing just a pair of Tommy Hilfiger jeans as people watched the circus from the other platform and the bridge. A train came, so I grabbed my clothes and boarded, but had left a trainer on the platform. I went to get it, but while I was on the platform, the train doors closed and the train pulled out of the station with all my clothes, my wallet and money (if I had any left). It was fecked up.

So, I walked over the bridge and out of the station barefoot and bare topped, wearing only jeans, and sat outside on some bollards in a state as the rain poured down. Three police cars turned up for crazy 'ol me and I was thrown into the back of one and bundled off to Tottenham police station and put in a cell.

I don't imagine I was talking much sense but somehow I'd given them some details of my parent's address, and one of the coppers recognised it as he was from my hometown, so they contacted them. I stayed in the police station for I don't know how long, with a rough woollen blanket to cover my torso and possibly saw a doctor. They gave me a cup of tea and I read the graffiti scratched into the walls of the cell, which was partly tiled, partly painted, with a small opaque window and had a toilet with no seat.

My father and brother eventually picked me up and drove me in torrential rain directly up to Manchester, where I saw a GP and was committed once again to the Krazy House, the secure mental institution. Holy Shit! Back at square one.

Here I was to stay for another six months, back on medication, again facing months of rehab and its guaranteed chronic depression, amongst other patients in similar frames of mind. This is not how I had hoped things would turn out, but here I was, in a worse scenario than ever: a lost, broken soul in a dire situation and a bleak outlook for the future.

When I left hospital I was given a council flat and I got by, minute-by-minute, hour-by-hour, day-by-day, watching the second hand on the clock, smoking Golden Virginia rolling tobacco through my stained brown and yellow fingers. Time went so slowly with depression that I'd go for a piss just to break up the monotony.

Alone in that flat has to be the lowest and loneliest time I have ever endured, waiting for the landline phone to ring, or the doorbell – a self-inflicted isolation with only cooking, shopping or cleaning on the agenda. Throughout all this, needless to say, my parents were a rock of strength, support and help, and I had occasional visits from a mental health nurse and made visits to a social worker.

I eventually gave up the flat as a couple of friends agreed to let me stay on their sofa bed for a couple of weeks in the living room, which turned into a couple of years.

It was better for me socially than the lonely flat I'd had previously, and I could only go to sleep when they'd finished watching TV and gone to bed, allowing me to crash on the sofa. I spent my days pottering around the house, listening to music and smoking. I often walked into town, shopping and looking in charity shops. I was soon back on the hash and drinking (but a little more in moderation) and ate regularly and started playing five-a-side football again, which I'd always enjoyed since a boy. This also helped me to keep in trim, great endorphins coming from sport and releasing frustrations of the trials and tribulations of everyday life. It also helped to counteract any possible weight gain that the medicine could cause as a side effect.

One night, while I'd just bedded down on my makeshift sofa bed, I heard a scratching at the window, so I got up and tentatively looked out through a gap in the curtains and there was a tall man in a dark hat with a screwdriver trying to prise open the adjoining kitchen window. Unsure of what to do, in a loud whisper, I called to Tommy upstairs, asking him what to do. He paused for a while and then said 'stick the lights on'' which I did and the wouldbe thief scarpered out of the backyard and down the alley.

Another day, I'd come back from town having bought a full box of Zig-Zag king-size, blue lightweight, rolling papers, and noticed a woman hanging about uneasily on the street corner, obviously a junkie. I thought nothing of it and went inside the house but soon started thinking something wasn't right. My suspicion and curiosity had been piqued and I looked out of the front window to make sure nothing was afoot. To my surprise, a man who also had the appearance of a junkie was shuffling down the street carrying a Dyson vacuum cleaner and met the woman I'd seen earlier. She had obviously been the lookout while her accomplice had broken into a nearby house. I immediately called the police and informed them of the situation, a robbery in progress. Now, any other capable thieves would have made a quick getaway, but this couple were so high and spaced out that they made little or no progress from the street corner and soon the police arrived and the two junkies were treated to a free taxi to the local cop shop at Her Majesty's expense. Bad junkies.

Another story involving a Dyson vac I enjoy retelling is when the sister of Pete, the man who owned the house where I was crashing, offered to clean our house. I think she was just being nosey and wanted to see the state of the place. Anyway, I came home one teatime and knew something was amiss as the carpets had been hoovered. I was the only one in the house to do any minimal cleaning such as washing up the pots in the kitchen when the fruit flies got too bad. Having a stranger come into the house made me felt uneasy and straight away I panicked about whether she'd discovered my stash of sensi. I'd left it on the mantel by the fireplace but it was no longer there. I asked Pete "where's my fucking weed!?" to which he just shrugged his shoulders and then I put two and two together and found the Dyson. Having a clear plastic barrel to collect dust and dirt was an advantage as I could clearly see the weed in the Vacuum cleaner. The daft cow had hoovered it up! Luckily, I was able to retrieve it and she never came to clean or snoop ever again.

Unbeknown to me, Pete's dad came round to fix the sink one day but I'd been blazing up the fire, smoking spliffs and bongs and listening to Kula Shaker's album *K*, reminiscing about India when there was a knock at the door.

I hid the bong under the sink and when I opened the door, a waft of smoke greeted Bobby, Pete's dad in the face. I let him in and imagine my delight when he said he was here to fix the sink. The bong was the first thing he found as he was tinkering with the pipes! Bobby later told Pete he'd seen me that day "zonked". Bholenath Mahadev Om Nama Shivaya.

I finally got a job in a pub in town, working four or five shifts a week tending bar. The pub was the cheapest in the town, part of the Sam Smith's chain, and attracted all sorts of characters, mainly an older clientele. The boss had been the British Army heavyweight boxing champion and was all ready to slap around customers who were looking for trouble, such as one drunken fellow who decided it was a good idea to start throwing potatoes round the pub.

Now the boss was very much anti-drug, but tolerated a group of drinkers he called "the druggies", as they were regular clients. They smoked joints outside the pub and took whatever narcotics in the toilets. I had to pretend I wasn't stoned when arriving for my shift even though I'd probably been smoking weed all day before getting to work. He would stress out if I was a few minutes late and say, "Get a grip, Breandán, get a grip!" I heard years later he had finally cracked, had a nervous breakdown and had attempted to commit suicide, not the first landlord to come a cropper on free booze. Get a grip, boss, get a grip!

There was a story going round in this pub, of a female dwarf who would offer oral sex for money to punters in the toilets, and her trick was that while in the act she would relieve the unwitting man of his wallet from his back pocket. I heard one day she was rumbled and got a good kick up the arse and never came back.

A woman who had gypsy or Irish blood sold cheap Golden Virginia, again off the premises at the door, as was the boss's rule. Some drinkers were definitely full time and arrived every day like clockwork. Each one had their favourite seat and would come in, put their coat on the back of the chair, slap the newspaper on the table next to a pair of spectacles, order a drink and sit down. It was as if they were getting into the office to start work, they had it off to such a tee. From their seat, they could get drunk; watch the horse racing and chain smoke cigarettes, as smoking was still legal in public houses in those days. The bookies was just around the corner, making it easy to place bets, and Saturday afternoon was a busy time in the pub as all the race meetings would be going off. The landlady served food – nice, cheap pub grub, so there was no excuse to leave.

At closing time, the boss walked his two dogs and rewarded them with a half a pint of beer each. I've never seen dogs age so quickly, poor things, they were around eight years old but looked double that. I never have been one to pass on weak human vices to animals, they are quite happy and better off without them.

I'd meet up with my friends when the shift had finished if they hadn't come in for a free drink earlier unbeknown to the boss, and go clubbing, spending my tips and having a laugh.

Daily life, though, was boring and unrewarding, and I felt trapped and depressed, looking for a way out. I'd been attacked a few times in broad daylight by aggressive people who wanted to vent their anger when I happened to be in the wrong place at the wrong time. I remember taking a nasty head butt on the cheekbone by a frustrated scally walking a toddler in a pram and a combination of punches to the head from an angry gypsy as I walked home with two carrier bags of shopping. When your luck's down, it's down. Such violence in whatever shape or form is to be abhorred and avoided if any creativity is to take shape and grow.

Well, after working six months without breaking a glass at the bar (which, to be honest, was seedy at the best of times but had been a rewarding experience for me) I'd saved up enough to return to India for the winter of the millennium. Yes, the call was as strong as ever and I was still hooked on the freedom I believe it gave me going there. I was adamant that I was going to learn from previous mistakes and not return to the psychiatric hospital ever again. I'd simply keep taking the medicine and avoid hard drugs. I was to avoid cities and stay around nature as much as possible, as the countryside fed my sensitive spirit. I was to distance myself from the rat race with its stress and pressures, and also from the stifling pressure to achieve and work from family and friends. Other like-minded friends I kept closer than ever and drifted away from others whose lifestyles seemed to be in conflict with my own.

17

INDIA AGAIN

Landing once again in New Delhi I felt born again, throwing off my straitjacket and shackled mind brought about by the confines of the mental institution. I felt happy with life, ready to savour another Indian adventure. I'd brought a guitar with me and frequented all my favourite locations. I spent most of my time in Goa, Gokarna, Hampi and Pushkar, and made a journey up to Kasol in Parvatti Valley, Himachal Pradesh.

In contrast to the sterile rigidity of a secure hospital and the rough, cold nature of a cheap boozer in a dilapidated, run-down northern town with all its aggression, factories and tension, I enjoyed this trip as much as any other, if not more so.

I made friends with some Italian guys who were funny, and we smoked and laughed all day long, first in Hampi and then at Om Beach. It was here I

117

first met the sadhu, Rocket Baba, on the familiar sands of this special beach.

A colourful character, Rocket Baba only drank chai, smoked chillum and ate a few hot chillies at dusk. He took me on as his 'Chela' (meaning disciple) for a while and we awoke every morning at five to salute Shiva and the stars, incanting Boom Shankar, Boom Bhole, Shiva Shambo, and fire up the sweet Malana crème in an Italian Alverman clay-fired chillum – monkey's breakfast!

"Have a rocket to the Milky Way," he would quip, as we blazed yet another chillum – his analogy that the pipe would transport or free one's mind, flying into the heavens, powered by the hit of the sweet charas chillum. He smoked profusely all day retiring around nine in the evening, ready to wake at five the next day.

Five in the morning is a very peaceful time in India with most people asleep, so you can focus on the stars, the galaxy, the heavens and the tranquillity of life, before India's hectic hive of action comes alive again at dawn.

He had a great insight into the mind and a deep understanding of Ayurveda, particularly in the use of the neem tree as a medicinal plant. Neem can be used as an antioxidant, a skin cleanser, an antiseptic, a lung purifier and general all-round immunity boosting tonic, also known as Margosa leaves.. Like me, his looks defied his age, begging the question that such a lifestyle, the charas or the *neem* or all three had an anti-aging effect, somehow slowing down the aging process and conserving the body, spirit and mind. Interesting uses here in the field of prevention of Alzheimer's.

I never saw The Rocket eat during the day, opting only to drink chai after chai and would only take five roasted chillies before retiring to sleep. He would often sleep in the cremation sights knowing there he would be undisturbed, as the majority of Hindus were superstitious and scared of such places.

I met up with Rocket Baba in different places around India including Pushkar, Kasol, Agra, Gokarna and Goa. His discourses were hypnotic and he was always the centre of attention. The local Indians were subservient to him and his caustic wit and intelligence. Some saw him as a charlatan, a freeloader and a scoundrel. For me he evades definition, he is sadhu, he is Rocket Baba.

A likeable rogue, rough diamond or mystic, Rocket Baba's charisma, charm and energy attracted fellow stoners such as me, and he could entertain a group of people for hours with stories, cutting comments and observations, in a truly theatrical, awe-inspiring manner. All this as we lit up chillum after chillum of pukka kwality and drank chai in beautiful peaceful locations like Om beach.

He taught me how to harvest and prepare the leaves from the neem tree in Pushkar and would direct me as to which branches to cut as I climbed the tree in this arid desert environment. We drank infusions of this bitter tasting leaf to purify the body and inhaled steaming vapours of neem to cleanse the lungs. It is described as the village pharmacy by villagers around India due to its many medicinal uses and benefits.

We shared a jackfruit in Goa, which is very large and

oval shaped, about 70 centimetres high and weighing maybe around six or seven kilos. Fresh jackfruit is delicious and a delicacy only found in the tropics with mangoes, papaya and lychee a ready alternative.

He would describe the trance parties as monkey parties and wish us well as we went to 'jump up and down.' He often referred to the Golden Age, referring to the 60s where he spent some time at Cambridge University.

We made a trip to Paradise Beach with my Italian friends, Rocket Baba and some beautiful German girls who were travelling around on an Enfield motorcycle. We sat around a fire on the beach at night, joking, smoking and telling stories, and the feeling, as ever, at Paradise beach was truly magical. I used to try and freak out travellers with my story of "The Shadow" – a blank panther that would allegedly pounce out of the jungle at night, surprising unwary prey, going for the jugular before dragging the unfortunate victim into the unforgiving darkness.

Later on, I disappointed Rocket Baba – I couldn't keep up with his ideals. I was enchanted by an Israeli girl I'd met, of Moroccan and Russian descent, called Tehila, which he didn't take kindly to and, in effect, he banished me from his sight and India itself.

Life was carefree but you had to be careful to avoid any imperial entanglements, i.e., the local police, as they were always on the lookout for foreigners with drugs. Such confrontations could lead to a prison sentence in a putrid Indian prison so it was to be avoided at all costs.

A policeman stopped and searched me in Goa and I was carrying a couple of acid tabs wrapped up in a rolling paper in a pouch of tobacco. He asked me what it was and I threw him a small Jedi mind-trick saying that it was just rubbish and I was off the hook. I wasn't always so lucky, though. Once I was in such a predicament in Goa as the police raided a chai shop restaurant ran by a French man and the cops found me in possession of Ich Tolla (ten grammes) of sweet Milana crème and had me in the back of the police wagon. It was night-time, and I was so stoned I fell asleep. Unbeknown to me, a fellow Japanese rocket star bargained my release, paying a baksheesh of 200 US dollars. I skipped town the next day to avoid any repetition of this situation.

The French owner wasn't happy as he'd already paid a bribe to the police that season so that the police would leave his establishment in peace.

18

ITALY

Keeping in contact with my Italian friends, I decided the best way to reintroduce myself gradually back into Europe was to fly from India to Italy instead of the UK, hoping it would be a softer landing and that I wouldn't end back inside the psychiatric ward yet again.

So, I arrived to the hills of Frascati surrounding Rome and spent a year on and off there. It was a lot easier to adjust to these friendly people, the lifestyle and culture, with many Italians having experienced trips to India. The Italian culture itself was at times quite laid back and they have an interest in alternative lifestyles. The Italians are very social people, and although they drink, they do so over lovely food, and the focus is on everyone enjoying a conversation and maybe some dancing, rather than getting extremely drunk and wrecked and out of control as I'd experienced in the UK.

The weather, with lovely blue skies, the mountain air and the diet suited me and, for one of the only times in my life, I actually put on weight, such was the food.

I taught a bit of English, went to a few Italian night school lessons and then worked in an open-air bar during the summer as a barman, which was thoroughly enjoyable. I had a few stories with Italian women and travelled around Italy visiting natural hot springs that were spectacularly illuminated in turquoise at night, and there we soaked in the pools with the steam rising up to the stars. I visited the island of Ventotene, the remains of an ancient volcano, which was idyllic with pure white sand in the Mediterranean with one simple fish restaurant serving locally caught fish. A popular Italian saying is:

"If you haven't eaten fish in Napoli, you haven't eaten fish."

Fabius, one of my Italian friends, a physiotherapist, happily showed me round these lovely sights and we would usually travel by motorbike, weaving this way and that. which was quite a thrill yet nerve-wracking at the same time.

Being in a new land helped me along, keeping my curiosity and spirits alive, subtly taking my mind off India and, at the same time, avoiding the depression of England and my Seasonal Affective Disorder (SAD) along with my destructive habit there of getting locked up.

I played five-a-side football regularly with

local lads and was rarely alone, with my hosts having many diverse and interesting friends and contacts.

I started chauffeuring for a man who had lost the vision in one eye after he was wrecked on drugs and booze and crashed his motorbike. He had been seriously injured as a result. I stayed with him in his home and drove him about whenever it was required, and his mum, who lived in the villa next door, prepared us sumptuous banquets of home cooked food twice daily. Unfortunately, I had money stolen from my room and was only working for food and board, but I wasn't sure who took it, maybe the maid or the gardener.

The man I chauffeured didn't work but rented out motel-type rooms by the hour to the ever-passionate Italians and their mistresses. This meant we had most of the day free to casually drift around, visiting friends, playing pool, drinking chai and normally ending up in the bars at night drinking. In fact he drank during the day, all day and every day. When he asked me to stop at the garage, it wasn't usually to fill up with petrol, but to drink a small appetizer called Campari, a red alcoholic beverage popular in those parts. It seemed strange that a petrol station would sell alcohol, but in Italy they do things differently. The art of coffee making, the barristas and cafés were immaculate, and customers would stand at the shiny, chrome bars, finely dressed, taking strong hits of café solo with a glass of water and maybe a cake and, no doubt, a cigarette. I smoked the brand Diana in Italy, a name that I found highly amusing, due to them having the same name of the Princess of Wales, who had died maybe five years before. All up in smoke!!

They liked to smoke in Italy and cigarettes were still legal in bars and public spaces during this time, and they had a penchant for sweet Moroccan pollen and Columbian cocaine.

I hooked up with a woman who was a coke dealer for a while and we had coke on tap, but although I used it for a few months, it wasn't really for me and I happily let it go. Maybe my medication dampened it's effects but it didn't bring the creativity or mystic high I associated with hashish.

One night I was driving through the cobbled, narrow picturesque streets of Frascati when a car careered down the road and bashed one side of the car I was driving and stopped abruptly. I got out of my car and approached the vehicle that had been driving hazardously. The driver, a North African, possibly Algerian, was obviously very drunk at the wheel and I asked him to exchange insurance documents to which he refused. He was acting rather strangely and to prevent him from driving off, I reached into the car to remove the keys at which point he bit on the arm. A friend called the carabinieri, the Italian police, who arrived in minutes and we explained the situation to them. Now the Italian carabinieri are pretty tough, with knee length shiny black boots, navy blue uniforms with a red stripe down the leg, and they carry pistols. They got the man out of the car and it became apparent he'd wet himself,, being so drunk. The police, disgusted at his drink driving or the state he was in, set about him by giving him a good beating with their truncheons. Rough justice.

The streets of Frascati were usually peaceful and taverns would sell the local white wine from barrels into decanters that clients would enjoy around simple wooden tables with red and white chequered tablecloths in the side streets on warm evenings. The custom was that friends would meet at these old establishments and bring delicious home cooked food and eat together lovely pastas, salads and strawberries washed down with cold Frascati wine from the cellar barrels.

Italians love to get together and talk, and every weekend they would meet at someone's house, to eat and enjoy themselves. In the summer, they would meet at communal barbeque areas in the countryside and pass the hot summer days drinking, eating and smoking and they enjoyed my guitar playing and songs as the sun set. When language is a barrier, I've always found music a good icebreaker and a way of communicating, as my Italian was very basic and I would lose the thread or find it impossible to keep up with conversations. I had a long skateboard, which I would walk up the country hill roads nearby and perilously fly down.

In the early summer, I recorded my first album at a friend's studio – songs I'd composed, and I was happy with the result. I paid for it by giving Simone a cheque which he never cashed. He wasn't the only one round here to live in a massive old villa, inherited from his parents, leaving him free to pursue his creative ideas. The album was called "At The Wheel".

At this time, email and apps such as Skype were revolutionising communications and I would go to an

Internet café to check my emails and talk online to friends. It was such a great means of communication; I used to keep in touch with the Israeli girl, Tehila, I'd met and travelled with in India. She lived in Tel Aviv, and we were in regular contact on the Skype messaging and video call service. We agreed to meet again so I boarded a plane to Israel in search of Love.

19

TEL AVIV, ISRAEL AND EGYPT

I was out of my depth in Israel; the sectarian tension that exploded into violence so often was only hidden under a thin veil. Strict codes of security were followed with bags being scanned for national coach journeys and armed soldiers were often seen here and there as it seemed the Israelis lived under a constant fear of attack, or paranoia of such an event. Suicide bombers on buses or at busy markets being a case in point.

I arrived to Tel Aviv airport from Rome, where Tehila met me and took me back to her flat. It didn't go well from the beginning as she'd been tripping on LSD the night before at a trance party and was out there. I don't know if I'd confused the form of the invitation but it wasn't as I was expecting. I ended up spending most of my time at the local beach where I met some musicians and we ended up jamming together in some studio. We smoked and drank a lot and Tehila was not best pleased that I'd smoked all her grass. Obviously I had no command of the language and people came and went from her flat and if they spoke Israeli, I didn't know what was going on. I met some recently drafted soldier, conscription being compulsory there for men and women, who didn't want to hold a gun and was under pressure from his superiors to toe the line. Not a good position to be in.

We made a trip to Jerusalem, which was uneventful. Feeling uneasy with the girl, I was just surviving the days with a broken heart, getting through whichever way possible. I didn't know what to do as I felt in the way at Tehila's flat, and it was very uncomfortable, so I decided to make a sojourn south to visit Egypt. I caught a bus to Eilat and then to the border and walked across the border between the checkpoints on my own. The crossing was heavily guarded on both sides with red and white barriers, turrets outposts and barbed wire, with soldiers patrolling each side, watching the other side warily.

I caught a taxi once I'd filled in the necessary documentation to the Gulf of Aqaba at the northern tip of the Red Sea, east of the Sinai peninsula and west of Arabia, with Jordan and Saudi Arabia to the east, with a permit only to visit this area, not Egypt as a whole. Dunes and tourist villages dotted the coastline but they were quiet of tourists, having had problems recently with terrorist attacks of which I was ignorant at the time. Close by was the site of the World War I Battle of Aqaba, led by Lawrence of Arabia.

I stayed in a small village with makeshift dwellings of wattle and palm tree leaf roofs, with a communal area overlooking the sea serving food.

The food was delicious. They served lamb shish kebabs, fresh humus and black olives, simple salads and local bread, covered with Nutella if you liked. They prepared tea and coffee and, there being a dearth of tourists, I was catered for very well. It was a strange feeling as the place was set up for hundreds of tourists but there were only a handful. I made a local connection to score some very rough grass that I smoked in a bong with a local young lad and we played pool and knocked about a bit. I smoked with a few of the locals who were peaceful and we also smoked shisha, a moist tobacco with different fruit flavours, apple and melon being popular.

One night Manchester United were playing Bayern Munich in Champions League, so we sat on simple wicker chairs round a small television outside a hut with some of the villagers and the local chief of police, watching the game and smoking shisha (Otherwise known as hubbly bubbly, hookah pipe or nargila) and pretended we were weren't stoned, out of respect for the Chief. Such is the pace of life in little villages like this where seemingly nothing ever happens.

I swam with a dolphin and its young and wandered the coastline, but my heart had been ruptured in Tel Aviv so I was just passing through time. After two weeks, I returned to the border, infuriating the taxi driver as I smoked the last of the grass in the back of the taxi. Some Muslims smoke cannabis and drink, some are dead against it – same the world over, whatever religion you choose.

So again I crossed the border and was interrogated at the Israeli side, as I'd been to a Muslim country, and this was not tolerated by the Jewish state. Stoned, I got through the questioning after being searched and had my visa cut from the original three months down to five weeks leaving me one week to leave the country. They questioned my reason for visiting Israel and Egypt, how I'd funded my trip, whom I was visiting and where I was staying and my sexual relations with any names I gave. Yes, I got a real grilling, and wondered what my Grandfather would have thought, who'd spent his life building and designing fighter planes, including during the Second World war to defeat the Nazi menace, which in turn freed the Jewish people and gave them this volatile Homeland.

So I shambolically continued up in Tel Aviv, and got wasted till it was time to escape this shithole.
I managed to go to a Trance festival the Bumbha Mela with Tehila and some of her friends in some dunes outside Tel Aviv at Hof Nitzanim. A trance festival celebrated annually on the Chol HaMoed Pesach, the intermediate days of Passover.

I was driving us both to meet her parents when we were stopped at an armed checkpoint and cautioned to proceed. I played football with her younger brother and we ate a meal together and I knew one word to say as grace was spoken, Shalom. Looking back, I'm glad I went, it was an experience I'll never forget and interesting how the heart can play with our emotions and thoughts and lead us on a merry dance.

So, being time to fly back to Rome, again I was interrogated at the airport and again I was stoned to get through it, pity the fools. I'd met some nice Israelis and some who were completely brainwashed paranoid fascists.

A lot of people get worked up by the situation in Palestine and hold strong opinions about it, or Gaza or Muslim countries from the comfort of their own armchair having never been to Israel or visited a Muslim country.

Good cop, bad cop – in the end its an on-going unfortunate conflict and situation, reverberating and causing repercussions worldwide.

It's easy to take sides, as millions hold one viewpoint of justice with millions taking an opposing view, which in turn just fuels the fire of further conflict, ingraining and inbreeding hate between nations which has existed for centuries.

Brought up with The Troubles between the United Kingdom and Ireland during the 70s and 80s, as a youth seeing tanks and soldiers daily on the six o'clock news, Molotov cocktail and stone throwing rioters against tear gas, water cannons and rubber bullets, I soon got tired of the mind games spun by governments and their lapdog media outlets.

It encouraged some people to join the British Army and others to contribute to the cause but I became very jaded by the whole affair of conflict, war, death and explosions. I just wanted an end, a peace.

Maybe this was down to the fact I wanted the world to be a happy, safe place for all, not an unreasonable ideology. Also due to the fact my allegiances were split having both English and Irish blood, I couldn't take a side and only saw the futility of constant fussing and fighting and its terrible bloody outcomes. No squabble, war or conflict anywhere in the world is any different; people take sides and seem willing to die on the basis of some grievance, maybe convinced they are doing right. My fucking hero.

This right and wrong duality has to be ignored, overcome and superseded and one has to find higher ground and accept things, for example, as in Buddhist teachings. Overcome twisted emotions and accept the illusory, temporary existence of what you believe to be true. It's not right or wrong, IT IS.

I returned to a similar life back in Frascati and was back and forth to Manchester.

Fabius came to London and I met him there for a few days and he visited me again in the North of England, I'd organised a trip for a group of people to go to a small village outside Keswick for a weekend, which I'd done regularly since my 21st Birthday.

These were always wild trips with about 25 people enjoying themselves in the beautiful surroundings this part of the world has to offer. The blend of mountains, lakes, forests and rivers with quaint unspoiled rustic buildings make this a very special place, with such natural beauty and geological formations. Dry stone walls and sheep are sometimes the only sign of man's presence here. To watch farmers and sheepdogs bring down herds of woolly branded sheep from the higher mountain pastures has always been a favourite of mine. There's something peaceful and ancient about it, man and dogs working in synchronisation and harmony and it's always left me in a state of wonder at the skill of such a feat.

We spent the time walking in the hills, through forests and along picturesque rivers in the day and walked two miles to the local pub in the evening. A friend tried smoking a chillum, but only managed to cough the entire pipe contents on the floor. It was not for him, being content with driving his Porsche and happy with his lot in life. Fair play.

I'd made some Fred Flinstone hash cookies which went down with mixed reactions, positive on the whole but, like a game of Russian Roulette, a couple of people found them too strong and had a rough one for a few hours.

A girl I'd known from Birmingham, who had also travelled in India, came as well and we had some fun together.

I'd tried surfing in Wales and Cornwall, convinced by a friend, 'The Stitch', I had to let the ocean into my life. It was fun and I enjoyed it and the longhaired, laid back smoking culture in harmony with the environment fitted me just fine.

When I was back in Frascati, some Italian friends were planning to spend the summer In Tarifa, the southernmost tip of Spain, overlooking Morocco, where the Mediterranean meets the Atlantic, and I too hopped on board, flying Rome to Malaga, via Brussels.

20

SPAIN

I'd hoped to surf in Tarifa, but actually it was a popular kite surf destination with constant strong winds called the Levant (Levante in Spanish) caused by its geographical location. A thermal wind that exists between Europe and Africa, moisture moves westwards along the Med from the Balearics until it hits the mountains between Algeciras and Tarifa. High pressure in the Alboran Sea and low pressure in the Gulf of Cádiz creates the wind funnel effect, favoured by the Rif-Atlas and Penibetic ranges, which create a strong 'Venturi' effect. Or, in layman's terms, it's always feckin' windy.

So, with too much wind and not enough waves in summer, I ditched my board in the flat I was sharing and went exploring the town and beaches.
The whitewashed buildings and quaint cobbled winding streets were very beautiful and gave some

shelter from the constant wind. On the beaches, one would get the full force of the wind and it was pretty unpleasant getting sandblasted by the wind and sand.

Most Spanish residents had already left to live in less windy places, but the ones who had stayed were driven half mad by the wind. Construction workers on scaffolding would be drinking beer by ten in the morning and shouting to workers below, above the noise of the gales. The void created by people who had left was filled by many travellers who came from different countries to Tarifa, Europe's most southern point where Europe met Africa and the Mediterranean met the Atlantic. There were many Italians who had come for the cheaper lifestyle, cigarettes and alcohol and hashish, as Morocco was just over the water. The hashish here was the cheapest in Spain and one could get top quality for a few euros a gram, a quarter of the price to be found in Italy.

I started busking on a small square in the evening where people would be sitting on bar and restaurant terraces and then going for a slice of pizza and drink in the bars and nightclubs. It really comes alive every night during four months of the summer with Spanish and foreign tourists looking to kite-surf, party or chill out.

A few miles out of the town were other less crowded beaches where hippies would set up camp in the forests and on the beach. Unfortunately, this area was restricted access and a military zone, and it was prohibited to camp there, so the illegal campers played cat and mouse with the Garda Civil. I stayed there for a few weeks, drinking sweet water from a spring and playing guitar with other like-minded travellers, snorkelling in the reefs and seeking shade in the forests from the 40-degree heat wave. Hashish could often be found here just lying on the beach, as currents lead here directly from Morocco and trafficers would deposit cargoes in the currents, hoping their merchandise would be picked up by contacts in Spain. Some travellers were into harder drugs and had an ugly habit of imbibing and then vomiting, possibly ingesting opium or heroin (known as caballo – horse in Spanish).

The police destroyed my tent on the beach, cutting it to shreds and breaking the poles, as I was unaware it was illegal to camp here, so I headed back in to Tarifa.

On the festival of San Juan it is the Spanish tradition to light fires on beaches while parties go on into the night. People drink alcohol around the fires with much celebration and music. I was drunk on sangria and when someone handed me a bottle of whiskey it seemed like a good idea at the time. I was soon very drunk and took a midnight dip with fellow revellers and then dried off by the fire.

21

MOROCCO

I had already decided to visit Morocco as you could catch a ferry from the local Port to Tangier, so with a bad hangover, I headed to the local scenic port and boarded a ferry to Africa.

I paid for my five-week visa on the ferry as it crossed the Mediterranean and had my passport stamped. Arriving at Tangier, I made my way to the train station and soon boarded a train to Marrakesh.

Marrakesh was a bustling, lively city with bazaars and winding alleys, busy traffic and the call to prayer sounding from the minarets of the mosques.

I stayed just off the main square, Bab Jamnafar, in a simple hotel and soon realised I hadn't calculated that I'd arrived at the hottest time of the year and it was 48 degrees! I needed to take a shower as I was sweating from just writing postcards.

One could find charcoaled braziers with sizzling lamb shish kebabs on skewers and other culinary delights in the bustling square at night, and Spanish, French, Arabic and English were all spoken by the market traders.

From Marrakesh, I headed west to the coast. to a music festival in Essaouira, a yearly festival attracting artists and music lovers worldwide. The main musical influence being Gnawa and fusion of this musical style with reggae and other genres. Gnawa is a typical Islamic music and can be described as a chant and its wonderful rhythms, melodies and beats can be hypnotic and trance inducing. Lutes and gimbris provide a distinctive Arabic eastern sound combined with the percussion of drums and the qraqeb or karkabas, metallic castanets that produce a sound similar to the beat of horses' hooves.

This usually sleepy fishing village and popular resort comes alive for the festival with free concerts and music happening daily and it's interesting to note Jimi Hendrix chilled out here in 1969.

I rented a couple of rooms from a man who offered me marriage to his daughter (which I politely refused) and made Moroccan mint tea with green tea, lots of sugar and fresh mint. The concerts were amazing and people had travelled from different countries from North West Africa to be here and the energy was electric.

I knocked about with a couple of local lads who showed me around the sights for a few dihrams (the local currency). I also gave them some surfing shorts, which they had taken a fancy to, and bought a rap mix tape off one of the boys who rapped in French and Arabic. One of the bands that rocked the

Kasbah was Gnawa Diffusion, an Algerian band that fused traditional African folk music with reggae and funk.

After the festival I hooked up with some travellers and we went a few miles south to Sidi Kaouki to play some music and camped out in a cave on the beach. Sidi Kaouki is another windy beach famous for kite surfing and wind sailing with constant, very strong winds. Unfortunately, I'd caught a fever with high temperatures. I had to sweat it out in a cave for days until the fever subsided, while my new North African friends played music and chilled out. The local 'Marquis' cigarettes didn't help, as they were very harsh and strong and give you a right cough.

When I recovered, I headed south in search of waves but it was the wrong time of year for surfing, with the best swells coming in winter. I arrived to Agadir and journeyed out of the city to Tagazout, another sleepy beach village. As I clumsily clambered down from the bus with my surfboard, a man ran up to me and happily announced: "There's no waves!" of which he was very proud, so I'd lugged the board all this way for nothing. Sod's law.

I hooked up with a couple of funny German guys who came here every year to ship local hashish back to Munich. I couldn't believe it, as the quality of the hashish to be found locally was terrible and mixed with God knows what, petrol maybe, it was an oily coloured dark green and smelt awful and toxic. They didn't seem to care and said they had no trouble selling it back home. One of the German men was furious as the receptionist from the hotel had robbed money from their room but there was little they could do about it. He kept shouting in a heavy German accent "vat is dis facking Bullshit!?" which I found hilarious. his friend, interested in Buddhism, took it in his stride.

We enjoyed meals of spicy prawns and fresh soft baguettes, washed down with café au lait, or café olé, as the locals quipped.

The Moroccans seem to have a knack for learning languages, probably due to the fact they are exposed to different idioms from birth. They have Arabic, French from Colonial times, and a lot in the north speak Spanish due to the influx of Spanish tourists. I met one man who unbelievably spoke Arabic, French, Spanish, English and Hindi, and was sat on a plastic crate in the street selling cigarettes loosely, one at a time. He'd learnt Hindi from watching countless Bollywood movies over and over again. Somebody with such linguistic skills could easily be a language professor at a university in the UK, yet here he was, eking out a living selling fags for pennies, or dirhams, actually.

From here I headed North to Meknes via Marrakesh as my visa was coming to an end. I was met at the bus station by a guide, who rented me a room, and here I stayed a few days in a simple dwelling in the city enclave, which was a maze of bazaars and markets and alleys. He had an Alsatian chained up, which was petrified of the huge cockroaches here, which would attempt to burrow in to his coat while asleep. I too was afraid of these cucarachas, which were the size of a fag packet and were horrible. I was taking a shower one day and one appeared on the shower door which

I nearly kicked off the hinges as I ran out of there. We smoked a lot and listened to music and had small parties with the locals. I gave some trainers to some lad I felt sorry for who had big cumbersome boots which I felt must be unbearable in this heat.

From Meknes, a local agreed to take me in to the Rif Mountains to the heart of the best hashish cultivation in Morocco; Ketama.

Here I stayed with a family of seven brothers on the agreement I bought a couple of ounces of top-quality hashish. In the evening, we all ate communally from a large plate of the local delicacy, tagine, using our hands and washed down with mint tea (thé de menthe).

Breakfast was in a makeshift café, which served as the local social centre, being the only place in the village with a TV. Here you could buy Danone yoghurts, coffee, tea and little cakes known here and in Spain as magdalenas. The locals amusingly liked to call them Madeline Albrights who, had been the first female United States Secretary of State, having served from 1997 to 2001 under President Bill Clinton who himself had been under Monica Lewinsky.

Ganja plants were everywhere here, irrigated from the rivers as the climate and landscape were very dry and hot and even the cockerels and hens were stoned here as they rummaged through the plantations in search of sustenance, inadvertently eating marijuana seeds and the like. The cocks, inebriated, would crow at any time of the day or night, seemingly not knowing or caring what time it was.

I was invited to play football with the local lads on a rough patch of wasteland but had to pay the privileged owner of the ball for the pleasure. We had a good game and a welcome shower afterwards to wash off all the dust.

The house I was staying at had a flat roof with bushels upon bushels of ganja drying out under the heat of the sun. They took a few of these and placed them on a wide-open drum with a special cloth and then covered it with plastic. Two boys then took turns to beat this with large sticks as if drumming, loosening the pollen from the stems and flowers, which filtered out into the drum below. This is the process Moroccan hashish is extracted to create hash, with the first beating being the beat quality and subsequent beatings obtaining a lower quality hash, or pollen as it's also called. One can test the hashish with a lighter and if it bubbles it is of high quality, sometimes known as double zero.

After a week in Ketama, I headed straight to Tangier as my visa was expiring. I was going through customs when an official called me over. I was stoned out of my face and after continuously smoking over the least five weeks in Morocco, it was coming out of my pores. He made a quick grab at a pocket on my leg, I think to test my reaction, but I didn't flinch. He asked me where I had travelled in Morocco and I said I'd been surfing on the coast, the board on my back finally paying dividends and he allowed me to proceed on to the ferry back to Europe.

I arrived in Tarifa, tired and relieved, but ecstatic that I had the best hash in town and hadn't been caught, and still had a few months in Tarifa to party it up before summer came to an end.

I had a liaison with a Brazilian woman and then got involved with a beautiful local girl but her father wasn't happy that this longhaired ganja smoker was fraternising with his daughter. Summer was coming to an end, and sensing that this girl could get me in to trouble as she was only 17, I reluctantly left town on a 24 hour bus, all the way diagonally across Spain, over a 1000 kilometres from the southern to the most northern province of Pais Vasco, The Basque Country, finally alighting in San Sebastian or Donosti as it's known locally.

22

THE BASQUE COUNTRY

I had visited Charlie in Zarautz, outside San Sebastian, during a few summers, staying on a local campsite enjoying a view of the beach that was popular with locals and tourists alike.

Surfing was a popular pastime here as it caught good swells from the Atlantic in the Bay of Biscay. The lifestyle was easy going and the Basque region was one of the more affluent in Spain, with heavy industry and munitions factories combined with a proud cultural heritage with its own language and customs.

John Toshack stayed here while he was the manager of Real Sociedad and he enjoyed the great diversity of culinary delights, the mountainous green landscapes complete with vineyards and apple orchards rolling into the sea. Having miles of coastline, the fishing industry is important here and

145

the delightful seafood on offer at the local markets
bears testimony to this.

I rented a flat with Charlie two minutes from the
beach and joined the local surf club and although it
took me a while to improve, I enjoyed surfing most
days throughout the year and had many a washing
machine experience. The local youth liked their reggae
and its surrounding culture, and hashish was popular
and could be seen being smoked openly in many bars.
The price of food, alcohol and cigarettes was
condiderably cheaper than in the UK, and the region
was booming, with money easy to come by.

I decided to busk here in the main
pedestrianized street near the food market and it
worked out well. My repertoire, mainly rock and roll
and English Indie suited the educated townsfolk and
I made a reasonable living busking here with my
guitar for several years. A typical day would consist of
busking, cooking, surfing and smoking strong hashish
in the bars with the Basque locals. They were always
friendly and polite although initially I didn't
understand either the Basque language or Spanish.
The level of English spoken here was poor and I
would go months without speaking English. Only
after listening to them having conversations in the
bars and shops for the first nine months without a
clue what was being discussed, did I start to pick up
Spanish. It proved easier to learn Spanish than Basque
due to my experience with Italian, another Latin
language, and my time spent in Tarifa. I wish I had
persevered with the Basque language (or Euskera) but
one new language was all I could handle at the time.
I'd been lazy at school and dropped French when I

got the chance, finding it taxing on my memory, which I still regret.

I slowly achieved fluency in Spanish or Castellan, not without the odd grammatical error, as I literally learned in the street. I picked up a smattering of Basque words and phrases, Euskera being an intriguing language, the way it sounds, how it is written and its history.

I started playing five a side football with some local lads and played tennis with Charlie, and I was given an old bike, which I got fixed so my life was very active and worthwhile. I had been given a new lease of life since those bleak, depressed rehab days and life was good.

Charlie would insist that I didn't smoke in the flat or even on the balcony, which I found constrictive and unfair seeing as I'd paid half the deposit on the rental. Luckily I spent most of my time on the beach front, busking or in bars.

I started to experience severe stomach pains and diarrhoea over a period of a few weeks and went to see a specialist in San Sebastian. Having analysed my digestive organs through an x ray with a barium meal, I was told I had a collapsed colon and the solution was to follow a controlled diet. I must admit, I'd been abusing my digestive system for many years now, with spicy and greasy food, alcohol, smoking, lots of bread and whatever took my fancy without paying heed to the consequences. Only recently in Tarifa, I had started drinking coffee and lots of freshly squeezed orange juice and my diet consisted of chocolate croissants, baguettes and raw chillies and pizza. It was a time bomb for my stomach and now it had gone off, quite literally.

The specialist was excellent and gave me a strict regimen to follow, which I still follow more or less to this day. For three months, I ate only rice, fish, apples and yoghurt and had a list of foods and products I was definitely recommended to avoid: pork, lactose, citric fruits, caffeine, alcohol and tobacco. I've never eaten pork since, quipping to the Spanish that I'm a Muslim and it wouldn't be kosher. Pork is the most popular meat in Spain, so much so that it's part of their national identity. When the Moors were settled here centuries ago, people would hang chorizo from their windows to identify their house as Christian.

The many ways the Spanish cure and present pork in the kitchen is seemingly endless; Pork chops, cured ham, salted ham, Serrano ham, chorizo sausage, salchichas and salchichon, fuet, pork lard – the list goes on and it is typical to be offered something containing pork as a tapas when you drink in the bars.

I chose to avoid lactose so that's cheese, cream, milk and butter, which makes eating out difficult and pizza a no-no. Nowadays there are many lactose-free alternatives to be found in supermarkets but back in 2003 the choice was limited or non-existent. To this day, I don't know if I had always been lactose intolerant but never properly diagnosed until now, because between the age of five and seven I stopped growing and despite numerous tests at the Hospital, the doctors couldn't find the cause.

I stopped drinking coffee, which is again a Spanish national pastime, and orange juice, but bypassed the restrictions on alcohol, just reducing my consumption a bit and continued to smoke. I'd been recently attempting to return to vegetarianism as I had practised in India but now my dietary restraints were so restrictive, I reverted to eating meat to give me a form of sustenance and nutrition. I wasn't helped as one day, busking in the street and trying to be vegetarian, an old woman brought me a hot steak in a baguette she'd just cooked for me and being hungry, it was too good an offer to refuse and back on to meat I went.

My digestive system more or less recovered but I've had a sensitive stomach ever since, not helped by the parasites I contracted in India and on-going stress.

One day while I was busking, a girl introduced herself to me, another musician who played the flute. We started a brief affair and she invited me to live with her and I accepted, not knowing that she was on the rebound after breaking up with a long term boyfriend recently and had been smoking a lot of skunk and not looking after herself. Within a month, she was in a psychiatric hospital. I'd left the flat with Charlie to live with her, and Charlie had since moved to Denmark so I was forced to rent a simple room with no heating or electricity, and access to a communal kitchen. It was basic but it did the job, although one winter morning, I awoke under a ton of blankets to a frozen glass of water by my bed.

I rented the room from a pensioner who seemed to go boozing and dancing every afternoon and if you tried to use the TV or hairdryer, the fuse would blow on all the electricity in the flat.

I took the local train, Euskotren, some days to other nearby towns to busk there and although it was a very good service connecting the towns and villages from Irun to San Sebastian and Bilbao, it had no toilet and sometimes I had to get off the train before my stop as I was called short.

I travelled over to Guernica and Mundaka by train as I'd met a man from here in Tarifa and would stay for a few days for a break.

In the summer, I would usually return to the campsite as I preferred to be outdoors, and I busked on a Dutch surf camp one year and gave concerts. The endless summers here were idyllic as one watched perched on a surfboard in the swells as the sun set over the sea, which would have a rosy, metallic glow, as if surfing in liquid Mercury. Waiting to take the last wave in, and then walk back to the campsite for some food and music beneath the stars are happy memories of this distinct region.

I worked one summer as a waiter on the beach promenade and had a side income selling hash or ganja. The cook, Mustapha, was Moroccan and we hit it off straight away. He liked his lager, cigarettes and cocaine whereas I preferred the hash. He'd spent his teenage years in Amsterdam and was very streetwise and after the bar closed around midnight, we would go shooting pool along the beachfront bars, which were always buzzing during the summer months.

Amphetamines seemed to be popular with certain youths but the physical damage it could do to one's body was frightening. I saw people in their 30s with bodies that resembled corpses.

The men were generally strong and active, dark haired and light skinned and had a great surfing level having being born into this environment, with eight year olds zipping along the waves with a skill level I could only dream of attaining.

The women were intelligent and beautiful, impeccably dressed and held a certain charisma, not unlike the French.

Winter would come and the tourists would disappear, as would work, and bars would close leaving the locals and a few hangers-on such as myself.

I rented a room with Mustapha, staying in a flat rented by some Venezuelan man who had come to study cooking.

Mustapha had recently got to know a Muslim girl as he knew her family and they had been dating secretly. She used to ring the bell early in the morning unbeknown to her father, and Mustapha would be snoring away, so I'd have to get up, let her in and then vacate my room while they had a bit of bedroom action.

The Venezuelan man was married but his wife was in Venezuela. He had a mistress, also from Venezuela, who he'd flown over to be with him. To his horror, his wife, maybe suspecting something, had arrived unexpectedly and unannounced, so he asked me to pretend that his mistress was my girlfriend. I'm a good actor. The guy's father apparently had a string of restaurants in Venezuela and was loaded, but he himself was a fat alcoholic who would fry chicken at night, half-drunk until a cloud of white smoke, a metre thick, would hang from the ceiling.

I got to know a Cuban guy, Dan, working in one of the chiringuitos on the beach who had trained as a dancer in his native Cuba but had married a Basque girl as a way of leaving his island and giving him his Spanish passport. His upbringing and education made him think in an entirely different way to Europeans and his views and perspectives on life were refreshingly distinct. He was a born survivor having withstood rationing and going hungry in Cuba, often joking he'd ate the neighbour's cat. He'd been well educated despite this and was an enthusiastic dancer and dance teacher.

This was my introduction to Latin Americans who came to work in Spain, in search of the good life in an attempt to escape the poverty back home. A number of the lifeguards or cooks and waitresses were Argentinian and were good company.

One thing that struck me though, was the number of Basque men who would travel to the Caribbean or South America and often return with a pretty, young woman in tow. Yes, sometimes these relationships lasted, but more often the case was that once the immigrant had found his or her feet and necessary documents, it would be adios amigo. One aged man in the town was famous for doing just that, bringing a Latin stunner home after every trip abroad, and after paying her way and setting her up, she would be off with someone else in the town. What a clown, but he was hooked.

I joined and trained with the local eleven a side football club and having long blonde hair, bleached by the sun and surf, at first they thought I was Columbian. It was funny as they were all in their early twenties and arrived to the training in their shiny cars, working, still living with their parents who cooked and cleaned for them while I was knocking 30, arrived on an old bike and had nobody to wash my dirty kit but yours truly. They were very friendly but the trainer was a bit more reserved and thought me an oddball and you could see the distrust in his eyes. Yes, I was a hashish smoking hell raiser but loved the beautiful game.

About once a year, I would visit Tarifa and old friends there, taking an overnight slow sleeper train from Bilbao to Malaga, which I always loved. It was great, going to sleep and waking up somewhere else.

One winter, I decided to stay a while in Busturia, in between Guernica (also known as Gernika) and Bermeo where I had an old acquaintance. Set besides an estuary, there was only one road in and one road out of this village and it seemed the only thing available to the young people here was hard drugs. Bermeo, a port, was a few miles up the coast and was a drop off point for narcotics coming in from merchant ships. I frequented Gernika and smoked hashish in the bars and played pool with the locals.

I eventually got a job as a plasterer's labourer and got some steady income for a few months while it lasted. It was hard and monotonous work mixing cement in the snowy hills outside Bermeo but we had a cassette player and one Alpha Blondy cassette tape I'd brought back from Morocco which we enjoyed listening to all day every day as we worked, sparking up the compulsory reefer. We would stop at one o'clock and eat in a local restaurant, wonderful home cooked food and reluctantly return to work later on.

With the wild plasterer, I agreed to go to Bilbao one Saturday night and he picked me up in his old Ford Sierra and picked up another friend called Kinky and off we drove to Bilbao. As we reached the outskirts of the city, we pulled into a park overlooking the bright lights and to my surprise and bemusement, they proceeded to jack up heroin. They removed their belts, cooked up the dose, flicked the syringe and injected their fix while I sat in the back. We then drove nonchalantly into Bilbao and partied it up for the next ten hours or so ending up at some after-hours club which was predominantly gay. I don't know if heroin increases your tolerance for alcohol but they could put it away that night while I got increasingly drunk.

The plasterer seemed to have an otherwise fairly normal lifestyle, was mostly jolly, working and had a kid. and somehow managed to keep it all together. Kinky was another story, lost in his world of music with a lot of ideas but never actually producing anything. His flat was depressing, with the obligatory cat and had a bucket next to his bed for when he vomited. The junkie life.

I shared a flat with Pedro, a fellow weed hound and Lamin, a boat engineer from Senegal. Lamin cooked a great spicy chicken and rice dish and was a nice guy although from a totally different clime and culture. His hands suffered in the cold here as he worked outside repairing boat engines but he worked hard sending his money back home to his wife and young child, visiting them only once a year for a few months.

Pedro was a different kettle of fish altogether who tried to survive by growing and selling drugs and doing odd jobs here and there. His girlfriend was a fat, coarse girl who somehow had got on local telly and was very arrogant and thought she was very special.

Pedro liked anything he could sniff such as coke or amphetamines and was having awful tooth ache and mouth problems in general as these caustic drugs caused havoc, destroying his gums and with all the alcohol and Coca-Cola, rotting his teeth. He had another bad habit of leaving his socks by the video recorder in the living room, his way of letting me know he'd been watching porn on the telly.

We got along at first but he had this cat that never left the flat. I've never been keen on cats as I'm allergic to them for a start but this one would destroy a packet of cigarettes in the blink of an eye if left lying around and was brought up to be a chain smoker. That wasn't so bad but it started to piss in my bed and it stunk to high heaven and was very inconvenient. The cat did it three or four times before I took a drastic step. I cornered the bastard and put it in a duffle bag and headed three kilometres up into the mountain and released it and denied all knowledge to Pedro on how his cat had disappeared. A few weeks later I saw it dead by a country lane, obviously run over by a car and I felt pretty bad and guilty about it.

When the plastering dried up, I started labouring for two middle-aged guys who were roofers. Again it was cash in hand and very welcome and on the strength of this, I bought my first ever car at the age of 33, a 12-year-old grey Nissan Sunny for

1200 euros off a friend of Pedro's. There was a story behind it, which I didn't get to the bottom of but involved some Belgian guy who was the previous owner who had split up with his girlfriend and something had gone on as he was currently in jail and the car had blood on the back seat and a broken window.

The roofers were real characters who would be in and out of the bar all day, boozing while working, snorting coke and smoking my joints. The boss wore a back brace as he'd inadvertently fallen off a roof and damaged his back on a previous job and I wasn't surprised, the way they were hammering the intoxicants. Not the wisest choice for someone in the roofing game. After we had completed the job, they hired a Rumanian instead of me who was probably twice as strong, so I took my car and returned to Zarautz.

I continued to busk, a local surfer family paid me to teach their daughter (who I now believe is an Olympic surfer) to play guitar, and gave some private English lessons.

I jammed with a band in Hernani with a Cuban Rasta called Raul and an Argentinian wizard, Juan Carlos, on electric guitar, banjo and mandolin. We had a few gigs but it never got further than that, though we had a good time jamming together.

One of the reasons it never got off the ground was the heavy drug taking and partying, which surrounded the group. They drank constantly and were always sniffing cocaine as well as smoking hashish whilst I preferred to drink black tea and just smoke joints. Several years later I found out Juan

Carlos had a stroke and whether this was down to his wild cocaine use, who can tell, but it doesn't help one's overall state of health, you can be assured of that. The stroke left him weak down one side of his body, which was a great shame as he was no longer able to play music like before. He's undergoing rehabilitation and only time will tell if he will ever fully recover but I'd say it's very doubtful. This is the price and danger one risks by overdoing the party scene as one day the body says enough is enough.

Another member of the band, Manu, recorded my next album "Chased Off The Planet" which I copied in Internet cafes and sold in the streets while I busked. The cover photo was a photo of a ganja leaf of the Himalaya a friend had sent me.

I remember visiting a girl in Northern France I'd met in Cornwall and en route I stopped at Hossegor to surf and spend the night. The next day, I smoked a spliff, put the shades on, put the pedal to the metal and carried on to drive north only to be stopped at a nearby roundabout by the officious looking gendarme who interrogated me and asked if I was carrying any drugs. The car was a mess with surf gear, empty fag packets and cigarette ends, food and camping gear. While two police searched the car, the other one continued to question me and I was baked after the joint but managed to keep it cool. They eventually found my CD with the ganja leaf cover and the gendarme asked me "What's this?" to which I replied "That? That's only music my friend!" with a big cheesy grin. They reluctantly left me proceed with my journey, having found nothing, the little bit of hash I was carrying was in the middle of a jar of lentils in a food box which they had ignored.

I did finally visit the girl in Normandy, but she was a nightmare coke user so I soon cruised back south through France and back to the busking beach-bum life in Zarautz.

I somehow managed to run the car and it gave me more freedom but sucked the little money I had. The years rolled by effortlessly in the Basque Country and one summer I had a holiday romance with a visiting Dutch girl from Amsterdam. It was the same summer I received terrible news from Ireland that a young cousin of mine had taken his own life after witnessing a traumatic shooting while on a year out with pals in Mexico, such a tragic loss of life, a lovely innocent lad with a great future ahead of him as a qualified pharmacist.

I had rented a room from a Brazilian guy who turned out to be very weird, not just the fact he'd had his stomach stitched in half, as he couldn't stop eating. I had a row with him as my money had gone missing and found myself again without a place to live.

I was missing the girl from Amsterdam who had returned home after summer, so I took a train to Irun on the Spanish French border and from Hendaya took a train to Paris on the overnight sleeper, walked across the Seine to another train station and caught a train to Amsterdam.

This completed a mammoth rail journey, albeit in separate stages, from Marrakesh to Amsterdam, a total of over 3000 kilometres. You gotta just love trains: Marrakesh to Tangier, Malaga to Bilbao, Bilbao to Irun, Hendaya to Paris, Paris to

Amsterdam.

We got on okay at first, the Dutch girl and me, but I was lost in Amsterdam, like a fish out of water after living in Zarautz by the beach. It also turned out she was still in love with her ex, so I eventually hitched a ride with a Dutch guy who ran the surf camp in Zarautz, back to the Basque country.

23

RETURN TO THE NORTH, UK

Again, winter had come, and I felt unsettled having lost my accommodation, lost my illusion of love in the Dam and lost my cousin in Ireland. I had the car, so on a whim I decided to drive home to Manchester and close the case on Zarautz.

I'd been there around five years and had become tired of not having a girlfriend so I thought I'd better try my luck somewhere else. My dad was upset about the loss of his nephew so I thought I'd show some support. Off I drove in my tatty banger, which pulled some 1.6 gasoline, going through France and crossing the English Channel in the Tunnel and then driving on the left with my LHD car with the old BI Bilbao number plate.

I stayed with my parents and again was unsettled to be back but got in touch with friends and landed a part time job as a peripatetic music teacher, teaching guitar in several primary schools around North Manchester. I was soon dissatisfied with my conventional role and battled with, depression using cigarettes to get me from one hour to the next, but teaching the kids was fun and looking back I enjoyed that even though I found the conservative nature and rigidity of the school system claustrophobic.

It made me realise I'm a rough diamond and feel alien in an environment where I have to pretend I'm something I'm not. I always seemed to be in disguise, wearing a mask, and everywhere I went was non-smoking, exacerbating my problems and perceived stress. Being a smoker in an office or a school back in the 70s was normal, but now it was shunned and looked down upon on, making the smoker feel like a leper or a criminal.

Anyway, I carried on but as always missed travelling and the freedom it brought. I retraced my steps to old jam nights and old dealer friends, so that kept me going and I eventually rented a nice flat nearby to my parents.

I had written some songs over the previous years while in The Basque country and recorded them at a friend's makeshift studio up in Yorkshire, a full album of my own compositions, which could be described as singer/songwriter blues. Writing songs helped me put a voice to my anguish, hoping it would bring out my blues and torment so I could advance to a better and more positive mental state. I was having trouble again smoking hashish, as it seemed only to bring me depression and paranoia. The album was called "Ride The Highway" with one of the songs being recorded in Zarautz with a surfer DJ friend

Makala. Pete Symonds, a great guitarist and Mandolin player put some great backing on the album and Mike Plummer at Rainbow studios added harmonica, noodling on saw and the Bass tea chest.

Pete had a similar infliction to me, often losing the plot and ending up in psychiatric institutions every couple of years as he didn't look after himself, forgot his medicine and led a chaotic lifestyle of couch surfing, but his downfall was he couldn't keep off the daily drugs and alcohol – he was his own worst enemy. So he continued to be in and out of mental institutions and the chaos that goes with it, known as a revolving door patient.

Luckily, I'd broken the vicious cycle of returning to mental hospital by taking the meds, eating regularly and being cautious most of the time with alcohol intake and avoiding hard narcotics, only smoking the weed. Yes Ma Lion.

I'd made friends with a recent arrival from Africa, Didi from Senegal, who had come at the behest of a much older English woman who'd met him on holiday there. Didi was struggling to adapt to this hard, northern clime and culture, getting drunk too often and losing his mind and cool. He played Djembe, a tribal African drum,, and we used to jam together getting wrecked on bad skunk. Years later I'm happy to know he's settled down, works in a warehouse, doesn't drink and follows a Rastafarian ethos and has many friends from his homeland and the Gambia in Huddersfield.

Skunk in the UK and worldwide, it has to be said, is

an aberration of the ganja plant, being way too strong for most people and almost toxic in the amount of THC it contains. One might as well smoke LSD. Mellow grass and sensi is hard to find these days and the demand for strong skunk has outstripped any other lighter weed and I'm not surprised by the consequential implications regarding the mental health of the young people who smoke it. But on a more positive and interesting note, currently with the advent of the Internet and more readily available information combined with increasing interest in medical marijuana usage, one can easily source ganja seeds with lower THC levels and higher CBD level strains. CBD buds can reduce the psycho-active components of the drug leading to a more mellow experience so the user can choose at the planting stage what desired effects he or she wants to attain. Such CBD strains can reduce the possibility of paranoias and panic attacks, serving only to relax the muscular system and the body of the host without heavy psychoactive trips or such undesired complications.

So just to look back and recap, since the diagnosis, I had battled to improve my physical, mental and economic state by bucking the system somewhat, unable to live in a traditional nine to five existence, using travel as a cure or form of escape. In this time since my diagnosis, I had achieved several notable strings to my bow since the initial bleak outlook, where I was unsure if I could just get out of bed in a morning and leave the flat.

I learned to speak and write Spanish/Castellan fluently, which is probably one of my proudest achievements since my breakdown. Many people struggle to reach a fluent level in a foreign language and I feel blessed to have this skill, but this wasn't obtained by luck but through patience, hard work, listening, being in the right place at the right time, making many mistakes but getting back up after each failure with a stubbornness that couldn't be beaten.

This is a paradox for fighting mental problems such as depression, as you have to uncover your fighting spirit which denies to lie down or be beaten, but to arise from each setback and to follow your chosen path despite the obstacles, and in doing so, achieving your personal goals. Your sense of freedom and liberation when these milestones are acknowledged confirm that at least part of your destiny lies within your own hands, thus giving life meaning and a purpose. Skin up.

I learned to surf to an intermediate level which was not only a great passtime, but guaranteed you were at one with nature, far from the madding crowd, the chatter and the traffic and such drudgery. Now I've tried many sports and regard myself to be a competent footballer, tennis player and skier but surfing was a whole new ballgame as there are so many variables in learning to surf, that it takes years of continuous practice to progress and the older one is, the more difficult it becomes.

But it was the call of the ocean that lured me in, already in love with nature and this sport had risk and adrenaline in copious amounts to stimulate and feed my troubled mind. Surfing focused my concentration, letting the mind settle, just me, the board and the waves. It also served as great physical exercise bringing welcome endorphins and giving my body a thorough work out improving the body physically through muscle enhancement, corporal flexibility and sweating out toxins and giving one a generally much more positive outlook on life. Any physical exercise or sport can do this, the advantage of surfing being that the seawater is a great tonic for the skin, and particularly for me, helped my complexion and soothed an otherwise itchy and dry scalp. On top of this, a good two or three hour surf session, however successful in terms of catching waves, I found to be a great hangover cure. It wouldn't matter if you got lucky and glided down some glassy faces twisting and turning at one with the wave or got tumbled about in the wipe outs of the washing machine wave, you would emerge refreshed and rejuvenated, ready to face the rest of the day.

Through honing my skills as a singer and guitar player. I became a competent performer of music, singing and playing guitar, recording several self-composed albums and performing concerts in different countries and settings.

Day in, day out, performing in the streets is live practice and my vocal chords and muscles strengthened, as did my confidence. This lead me to playing in bars and playing in various bands which was helpful socially and artistically, allowing me to nurture, develop and pursue my creative capacity which is necessary for any artist. Music doesn't have a language or fixed frontier and can help grease the cogs when people of different races, religions, mind-sets or cultures meet, fuse and eventually become one. The fact that I was a poor wandering minstrel, with long hair and an attitude and dress code to match, allowed me to open doors to places and people that would have been firmly closed to a rich man attempting to repeat these experiences. Being a troubadour on the streets of a foreign land gave me time to observe the people and gain a perspective on their culture, what made them tick and to fine tune my skills of character assessment by examining all aspects of a person's being from outward signs such as dress code, posture, confidence of gait, body language and the image they portray at a given time and place.

If I walked into a bar of 80 people and said to you that in four minutes they would be all clapping and whistling and feeling elated, you may ask what love drug I was planning on to administer. Yes this drug is called Live Music played from the heart and conveying a definite message, with each concert having to be pitched correctly to the audience so that the majority of them enjoy it and take and experience a part of you with them for a while.

Performing live can be deemed a type of hypnosis or brain washing and when you have the audience in your hand for a fleeting moment, it is wonderful and should be handled with the utmost care, sincerity and respect as you guide your albeit temporary followers to a temporary destination which is the dream the song conveys. For example, this may be a state of love, melancholy, an obsession or addiction, blues, the beauty of a lover, a drug induced high or vision, a sense of despair or a broken heart.

Composing and performing music is active meditation and at the same time a cathartic process as one self-analyses one's own situation, thinks about it, remembers and feels it, puts it into perspective and records it, first on paper, then music is written to match these feelings or occurrences giving it a real physical existence. Changes are made initially as the overall picture becomes clearer and finally the song has taken shape and shared with listeners and recorded in whatever format. The song now exists as a part of you but now separately from, apart from you. This allows the writer or experiencer to see his own experience from a third person perspective, it allows him to be free to forget the experiences as it is now recorded for future reference in a written, digital or CD format and thus enables the writer to advance and progress on to new avenues of life and therefore new material. The initial pain or pleasure or feeling that drove or inspired the writer to write the song will dissipate quicker due to its exorcism from the mind and being shared with others.

Let's go back to that word cathartic, as I find its definition useful to clarify what I'm attempting to explain:

Providing psychological relief through the open expression of strong emotions; causing catharsis.
Synonyms:
Purgative, purging, purifying, cleansing, cleaning, releasing, relieving, freeing, delivering, exorcising, ridding.

I'm stressing this point because I found creativity and works driven by it, whatever its perceived economic or academic worth, to be absolutely essential to the artist for his mental and spiritual wellbeing.

Crying is a cathartic release available to all, yet so is abstract painting, graffiti or mural painting, writing, composing, designing or singing.

When a person who is of a creative mind ceases to create, it causes stress, anxiety and frustration and will, in turn, create an imbalance in the soul and the person's mind-set.

All our experiences so far in life go into that brushstroke, word or note and if we only absorb experiences but don't put pen to paper we become mentally blocked. Such is the world today with a constant overload of information, it is vital one learns how to channel all this into a creative, positive, worthwhile output. It's like a funnel where we take everything on board through our senses, drop the information regarded of being without merit, sometimes blocking out information we deem as frightening or unhelpful if necessary, and channel the rest into an output. In doing so you have processed the information taken on board and synergising it all, have created something else, that although is recycled is completely new. A true artist should reflect on how they feel in their work, or it is worthless, a fake, easily copied and forgotten.

Some friends of mine in Madrid got in touch and asked if I could help out a girl they knew who wanted to come and study and work in Manchester. So I agreed and met Lucia at Oxford Street train station, one summers day. The rest, as they say is history.

We got on well and I managed to get her on some basic English college courses in the local town, as her English was non-existent. We'd chatted online and I thought she had a rudimentary English level but she'd been using an online translation app to understand the conversations.

It was summer, so we took the ferry to Ireland in search of Guinness and waves, still in my Nissan Sunny, which now had English plates and went camping down the west coast of Ireland. Even though it was the height of summer, it poured down with rain every day and was freezing but we had fun and the landscape was beautiful.

I surfed on a few beaches but one day inadvertently stood on a weever fish, which was very painful for a while and left me out of action. They eject a strong venom into the sole of the foot through spikes, which can lead to temporary paralysis of the affected area.

We camped, sometimes rough, in pine forests, making smoky fires at night and sometimes pitched on local campsites to enjoy the hot shower facilities. Lucia was quite wild and I had to curtail her penchant for shoplifting as it did my head in, she soon stopped after remonstrating with her and after she had had a few close calls with security personnel.

She was very bubbly, energetic and enthusiastic, Manchester all being a new world to her and she thrived at studying, now at a college in Manchester. She began to work part-time in a Pret a Manger which was like the League of Nations with all the different nationalities working there, so she fitted in just fine while improving her English.

I started seeing an old school friend who also had a Spanish girlfriend he'd met in Dublin so we could have made a good coupling but unfortunately he had a lot of trouble with the drink. Being alcoholic, his mood swings and behaviour were unpredictable and he rarely drank in pubs, being banned from many, preferring to drink at home. I tried to get him out and encouraged him to join the jam sessions as he was a talented pianist but he was tied to the off licence and strong liquor. He had a good job as an accountant but slowly but surely through drink and a series of bad decisions, he lost it all.

His girlfriend left to Spain, then not long after that he lost his job, seemingly preferring to spend his time drinking on park benches with local down and outs and junkies. He crashed his car while drunk and was lucky to escape unscathed and finally lost his flat. From a cosy life to homelessness on the streets of rage within six months or so, he contracted meningitis, was induced into a coma and now he's still picking up the pieces with his health ruined and a very bleak outlook facing him now.

Alcoholics are difficult to deal with as it seems a never-ending circle of catastrophes and unlikely that they can get off the drink and the damage they do to themselves and loved ones. They serve to the rest of us as a reminder of the dangers of drink. Luckily, my hangovers are so bad after drinking that this alone keeps it in check for most of the time.

Lucia and I were quite happy for a time and her English improved. She was easily likeable, being young, funny, happy, enthusiastic and outgoing.

Being a city girl, she tired of the village and convinced me to move into inner city Manchester, a stone's throw from Moss Side where it would be an easier commute for her and more lively.

The terrace was old and drab but we made it

homely and I ventured the streets joining a few local jam sessions and got my guitar singing at a local Rastafarian Community centre on Claremont Road, Rusholme.

I felt the vibe on the street a bit intimidating and didn't like to go out walking at night, but we were close to the city in this multicultural area. We were near to Asian food wholesalers and Hubbly Bubbly Sheesha cafes which I frequented during the day, whiling away the hours. The curry mile was just next door so a good curry was easy to come by, but my favourite place to eat was at the This n That in the Northern Quarter down a rundown derelict back street. There were several similar eateries in this area with good cheap, wholesome spicy food and soft chapattis.

After work, I usually stayed in and listened to music, cooked the dinner and waited for Lucia to come home. The cold weather, hard attitudes and the fact that she missed her native home, friends and family were slowly chipping her lively spirit away. The food, culture, language and nightlife were difficult for her to get used to and, after two years in Manchester, she'd had enough and longed to return to Spain.

I'd been in a similar boat in Manchester, felt out of it, just surviving financially and always bordering on depression, smoking tabs to get me through the day and smoking hash in the afternoon and evening to put up with the boredom. Friends had their own busy lives and I saw them infrequently, usually in the city in a few pubs and clubs.

The traffic was busy and hectic and I found it draining commuting an hour to the schools and spent as much time driving as I was teaching. The personas of scallies in tracksuits hanging around outside convenience stores put me on edge, not knowing if an aggressive confrontation was on the cards.

So, I had to make a decision: whether to stay in Manchester or return with Lucia back to sunny Spain.

It was a no brainer really – after many years without a partner I had to try a new life with Lucia, back to a country and language I knew well.

We decided not to move to Madrid but to Galicia, a rural, green part of Spain in the north west above Portugal, where Lucia's father owned an old farmhouse built in 1840, which had been empty and dilapidated for many years.

So, with my car packed to the brim, we set off on the journey to pastures new, going south from Manchester, past Birmingham, around London until we reached that marvellous feat of engineering, the Channel tunnel which took us under the English Channel to Calais.

From Calais we drove south, south-west, stopping over at a French bed and breakfast for the night to get some welcome rest. The motorways in France were fairly free of traffic but the tolls amounted to around 100 euros.

The next day we crossed the border at Hendaya /Irun and entered Spain where we stopped for a picnic on the beach in Zarautz, outside San Sebastian. This was familiar territory to me, having spent five years living here. We then traversed the northern part of Spain, passing Bilbao, Santander, Gijon and Oviedo.

It was night-time when we arrived in Galicia, our final destination. My backside was sore from almost three days' driving but my Citroen Xsara 1.6 petrol had served us well. With no GPS and only a map to guide us we were happy to have arrived safely and in one piece.

This was a region of Spain I'd never visited, but I hoped to leave my melancholy behind in Manchester and start afresh once again in the Celtic land of Galicia.

EPILOGUE

The Galician landscape is beautiful, green and lush, but the region has often been neglected by the capital, Madrid. It has its own particular language Galician, but Spanish is also widely spoken. It also has its own traditional culture and cuisine and has similarities in weather and topography to Wales and Ireland.

There is none of the bohemia I've experienced in other parts of Spain. The region is a traditional farming community, like rural Ireland 60 years ago. You can often see old women working in the fields, tending cattle and chopping wood. Galicia as a whole has been a poor and sometimes backward rural area with limited investment into its infrastructure, so that many people here over many generations have had to emigrate in search of work and better living conditions.

I'm currently living at 450 metres above sea level,

where the land is saturated by precipitation during the autumn, winter and spring and then baked dry in the summer. The land is, at times, boggy, swampy, marshy – a type of moorland where pastures for grazing have been farmed for centuries and forests of oak harvested for firewood. Chestnut trees have provided timber for construction and furniture and the old bullock-drawn carts. The chestnuts, in abundance, were and still are a welcome form of sustenance in the autumn.

There is cattle farming here for both milk and meat, and most rural abodes have their own allotment for vegetables. Most rural houses in the communities are still very traditional and partly self-sufficient, rearing pigs, rabbits, hens and chickens alongside larger bovine and porcine livestock and sometimes apiculture. The pigs provide famous delicacies of the region including chorizo, Lácon, salchichas, fuet and jámon (ham).

To be poor in a rural setting where one can rely on the beauty of the natural surroundings is far preferable to being poor and captive in a concrete jungle with all its aggression, undying pursuit of materialism and 'bigger is better' mentality.

The slow pace of life suits me, leaving the stress of the city far behind. Despite this, rural life brings its own set of different challenges and adventures but, at the same time, it's rewarding, being in harmony with nature.

The twists and turns of life have so far have been varied and colourful and as I slow down, I'm pretty content with how things have turned out, despite the ups and downs.

India, for me, remains a constant source of inspiration: rejecting the commercial and the mundane and replacing it with the colour and energy that I experienced there, the freedom, the dramatic landscapes and the pulsating energy.

Having had the chance to travel and live an alternative lifestyle has brought me untold rewards and a fair few mishaps and, like a pinball in a machine or a leaf in the breeze, I'm glad I've ended up where I am today: in the countryside, surrounded by forests, weathered by the four seasons, far away from the madding crowd.

Nowadays, I tend to respect alcohol and attempt to drink in moderation, as infrequently as possible. After smoking hash and ganja for 30 years, I have slowly let it go, smoking only self-cultivated CBD marijuana for a few years and recently stopping it altogether, only smoking organic blonde tobacco. Mental illness still provides a constant challenge and complicates life, but through various coping strategies and a rural lifestyle, I have found it easier to confront my demons.

ABOUT THE AUTHOR

Breandán Ó Seighin is a creative aura of energy now residing at altitude in the Galician countryside in North West Spain. Having completed a formal education, he travelled extensively around India, walking in the Himalaya, frequenting tropical beaches on the Arabian Sea and travelling over 6,000 kilometres on public transport there, always with his pipe and hashish.

He has busked in the streets of the Basque Country, chauffeured in Italy, played football in Italy and Spain and the Rif Mountains, smuggled contraband between continents, surfed in the Atlantic ocean, played countless live concerts, travelled by train from Amsterdam to Marrakesh and despite being locked up a few times, has learnt how to survive with schizophrenia.

Printed in Great Britain
by Amazon